DATE DUE

GAYLORD			PRINTED IN U.S.A.

Outside

FITNESS

A Comprehensive Training & Nutrition Guide for an Active Lifestyle

PAUL SCOTT

Foreword by Chris Carmichael, U. S. Olympic Committee Coach of the Year

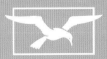

W. W. Norton & Company, Inc.   New York   London

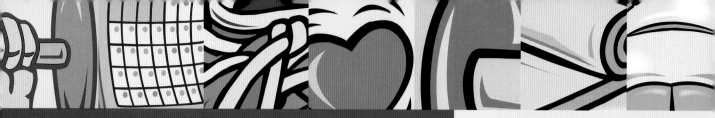

Some of the material in this book appeared in a slightly different form
in *Outside* **magazine and** *Outside Online*

Library of Congress Cataloging-in-Publication Data

Scott, Paul, 1963–

    Outside fitness : a comprehensive training & nutrition guide for
an active lifestyle / Paul Scott.

    p. cm.

Includes index.

ISBN 0-393-05971-5 (alk. paper)

    1. Exercise. 2. Physical fitness. 3. Outdoor recreation. I. Title.

GV481.S34 2006

613.7'11—dc22

                             2005045408

Front cover photo © Ron Chapple/Getty Images

Back cover photo © Jorg Bardura for stocklandmartel.com

Cover design by Johnson Design, Inc.

Interior design and composition by Carol Jessop

Illustrations by Mike Biegel, www.mikebiegel.com

Published by W. W. Norton & Company, Inc., 500 Fifth Avenue,
New York, New York 10110

Printed in China by R. R. Donnelley

10 9 8 7 6 5 4 3 2 1

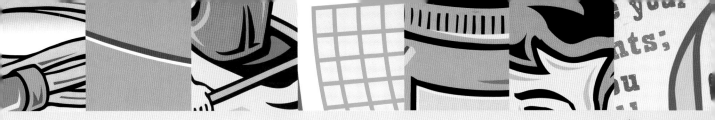

A DISCLAIMER

This is an advice book about training written by a writer, not a professional trainer. The advice given is meant to facilitate a reasonable level of self-directed training, but this book is not, however, a substitute for those areas of fitness where a personal trainer or coach is recommended. These areas include, but are not limited to, the methods of power, strength, yoga, balance, and agility training offered in this book. Nor is the advice stated in these pages meant in any way to be taken as a substitute for professional medical advice. Always get permission from your doctor before beginning a training program, especially if you have a history of asthmatic, respiratory, orthopedic, or cardiac problems, sports injury, or a family history of heart problems. Training is individual, and any one workout may not be right for all persons. The author and publisher disavow any and all liability from injury resulting from the methods written in this book.

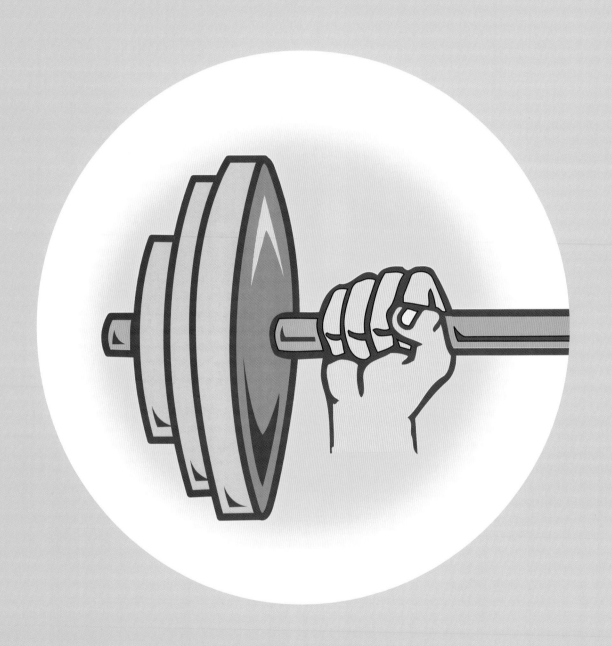

CONTENTS

ACKNOWLEDGMENTS

In reporting for the articles that helped inform this book, it was my good fortune to interview the following talented and generous researchers, trainers, fitness entrepreneurs, and athletes: William Kraemer, Beryl Bender Birch, Jay Blahnik, Tudor Bompa, the late Ed Burke, Chris Carmichael, Ed Laskowski, Jay Smith, Jimmy Radcliffe, Don Chu, Joe Friel, William Ebben, C. C. Cunningham, Dan Benardot, Nancy Clark, Edward Jackowski, Eric Harr, Ed McNeeley, David Musnick, Al Vermeil, Vern Gambetta, Paul Chek, Juerg Feldmann, Steve Myrland, Roy Simonson, Andy Walshe, Scott Benson, Terry Laughlin, Jeff Galloway, Peter Reid, Tim DeBoom, Peter Lewis, Mark Tarnopolsky, Jim Rutberg, Mike Clark, and Steve Ilg. There were others, but space is short.

Training is home to many disagreements, as well as proficiency far greater than I surely possess, so I am certain that some of the individuals mentioned above may differ with some of the advice contained herein. As such, anything I present well, they can take credit for, and any errors are of course mine. I have worked carefully to present this material accurately, but experience has taught me that an exhaustive look at a field of study on the part of an attention-deficit magazine writer will surely give rise to an occasional error. I am especially grateful to those individuals who previewed advance portions of the manuscript for accuracy, including Joel Friel, Jim Rutberg, William Kraemer, and Steve Myrland. I am also indebted to the people at Human Kinetics Press, whose books have presented such a reliable source of well-researched training information, and whose publicity department graciously provides them for reporting.

The idea for the "Shape of Your Life" series that gave rise to this book was suggested to me by Nick Heil, my fitness editor at *Outside* for many years, who also edited early segments of the series and guided it toward more inclusive, plain, and inspirational language each step of the way, a contribution my writing surely requires. Major contributions in the editing and creation of that series were also provided by Chris Keyes. The people at Away.com, the administrators of *Outside* Online, let me try my hand at answering fitness questions online for which I am grateful if still a little stressed out by the experience. Portions of this book appeared first as my answers to some of those questions, and other portions first appeared under my byline in *Outside* Bodywork over the past six years. As such, the writer would like to thank everyone at *Outside* as well as editor Hal Espen for continued support. The writer would also like to thank John Barstow, Kermit Hummel, Jennifer Thompson, and Julie Stillman at W. W. Norton; and Bill Contardi at Brandt & Hochman. Thanks finally to my wife, Leslie Sim, who has always been my foundation of strength, humor, and support. She let me fill up our small one-bedroom Wicker Park apartment with stability balls, dumbbells, yoga mats, and all sorts of training stuff.

FOREWORD

My career as a competitor and a coach has its roots in cycling, but truth be told, pure cyclists are not very good athletes. As Lance Armstrong's coach for more than 15 years, I can tell you that one of the keys to his longevity was our focus on keeping him active in a variety of sports and activities.

Lance started his athletic career in triathlon, and became a professional by the time he was 16 years old. Yet, even though he made the transition to full-time cyclist two years later, he never truly gave up his running shoes, or his swim trunks. For that matter, he never gave up basketball either, and his competitive side has never been able turn down a backyard pickup game—of anything.

The human body is an amazing machine, capable of completing a wide variety of movements and functions. Yet, when you limit its functions by specializing too heavily on one sport or type of exercise, be it running, weight lifting, or any sport that involves repetitive movements, you not only limit your ability to participate in other activities, but you also limit your ultimate potential for success in your primary sport.

By using his body outside of cycling, Lance improved his performance on the bike and reduced his risk of injury at the same time. In fact, during the course of his long career, Lance suffered very few injuries. Sure, he lost a lot of skin in crashes, but he didn't have to endure lasting problems with tendonitis, muscle imbalances, poor flexibility, or brittle bones that can plague a professional cyclist's career. As a result, Lance was able to complete more days of quality training, which was a critical advantage in his preparations for the Tour de France.

Having a well-rounded base of fitness is as important for everyday life as it is for athletic performance. Paul Scott has it right when he talks about the importance of developing functional strength, endurance, and agility. These are the capacities that allow us to lift our children without straining our backs, play in the company softball game without pulling a hamstring, sling a pack onto our backs for an impromptu weekend camping trip, and take part in local charity runs and rides without fear of injury or excruciating pain. Being a complete athlete means you have more options and more opportunities to have fun and explore new possibilities. The world is outside, waiting for you, and this program can help you make the most of it.

—Chris Carmichael, U.S. Olympic Committee Coach of the Year

INTRODUCTION

The American Way of Fitness

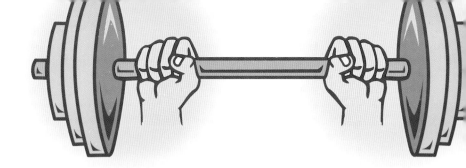

If **MODERN FITNESS** seems out of sync with the goals of simply becoming more effective and versatile outdoors, it's because fitness is still a **RELATIVELY NEW PHENOMENON.**

Studies may populate exercise-science journals, but aside from the narrow utility of research that helps elite performers achieve greater heights, it is hard to get away from the sense that the entire fitness industry came about because of the disappearance of domestic and farm labor. The basic movements we had evolved to practice day in and day out have all become automated, and our bodies are paying the price.

Look around your home. Your clothes dryer replaced a daily workout required of your great-grandparents, who needed upper-arm muscular endurance to operate clothes wringers and the back flexibility, muscular endurance, extension strength, and core strength to pin a load of wet wash to the line. Your six-burner stove eliminated the need for the upper-body power required to split a cord of wood. Your ATV erased the daily endurance workout needed to ski to town through a fresh dump of spring snow. Your car's seat back eliminated the core strength needed to hold yourself upright on a horse.

Your power mower and snowblower replaced workouts filled with pushing, bending, rotating, and lifting, and today even manual laborers have seen the squatting, lifting, rotating, and throwing become automated out of their lives. The city crew that just took down my elm showed up using bucket loaders to throw the foot-wide stem portions into their truck bed. If they want to be able to squat, lift, and throw, now they have to go to the gym after work. The gym—where they learn to walk up stairs while leaning on their elbows, push weights from their chests while laying on their backs, and build lots of odd little muscles best used for show. Is it any wonder we forgot how our bodies actually move?

BODYBUILDING:
THE CURSE OF ARNOLD

Most gym work today evolved from a practice known as bodybuilding. Bodybuiling, of course, was popularized as a way to better define and enlarge your musculature. You build muscles through *hypertrophy*, the term for overloading a muscle to the point where its fibers break down and subsequently become enlarged. You may need to move weights with complex movements in the real world, but most hypertrophy is achieved in the course of moving heavy weights very slowly and in very specific, isolated, and limited contexts.

Both strength and hypertrophy are developed by the progressive addition of weight to a barbell, yet this overload is made possible largely through placing your muscle in an artificially created context of isolation. At the gym, the benches, arm rests, pads, and chair backs aren't there to warm up the place—they artificially shore up the muscles being targeted, building little exoskeletons around them to take the place of your own, not-so-strong anatomical support structures. The typical curling bench is a fine example of a way in which bodybuilding gets you strong at unrealistic tasks. Because you are resting your arm on a support beam, basically causing the strength of the support beam to substitute for defi-

cient strength in the muscles behind your biceps, your artificially enhanced support muscles (in this case, your triceps) no longer limit your target muscle (your bicep).

Isolating a muscle like this enables you to challenge it far more than it could be challenged in a natural context, which is why there is always a role for isolated muscle building in building basic strength. For the untrained, atrophied American (that would be most of us), you can benefit from first building muscles in isolation before building muscles in the collective groups in which they actually are used in everyday work—especially if it is an increase in muscular size, rather than strength you are after. For the beginner, it can make sense to push a weight on a machine press for a time before you do the same movement with a push-up, before you do a bench press, before you do a standing cable press—four forms of the same basic pushing movement, but only the last one helps build strength that most resembles how you will use it once you get outside the gym. Indeed, some trainers make a good case

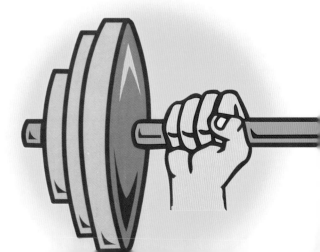

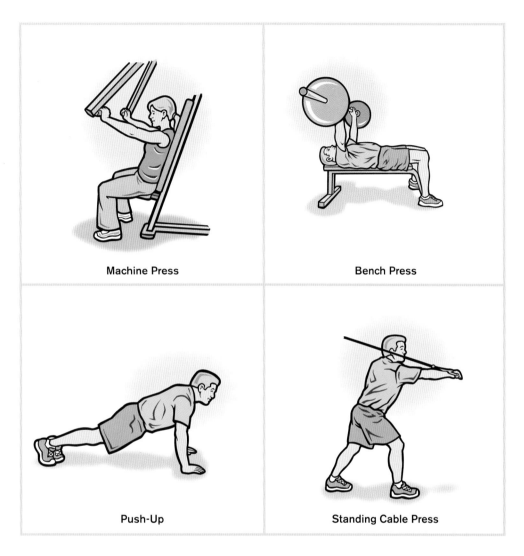

Machine Press

Bench Press

Push-Up

Standing Cable Press

Machine press, bench press, push-ups, and a standing cable push; all pushing movements, all useful, but only one resembles how you actually push in real life.

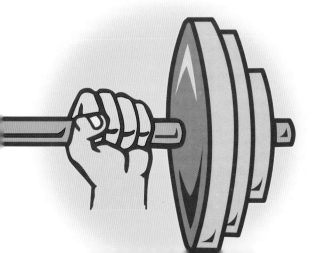

for starting only with modified versions of body-weight exercises before ever picking up a dumbbell. But in their focus on overly supported or one-joint movements, gyms can teach us to stop our progression before getting to naturalistic movements.

Few naturalistic movements—especially those on the trail, the field, the river, or the rock—involve flexing just one joint sitting on a chair or laying on a bench. Usually the real demands we face require so-called integrated or *multijoint* movements of the ankle-knee-hip, or shoulder-elbow-wrist variety. More often than not these real-world movements include both *closed kinetic chain* movements, where the chain of force terminates (is closed) at an immovable point, such as the ground, and *open kinetic chain* counterparts, where force is redirected into some moving apparatus such as the swing of a leg. The value of working in both closed and open kinetic chain exercises sounds academic until you consider the fact that nerves control your muscles, and that pushing something mobile teaches your nerves a different lesson than pushing something immobile.

The simplest bounding movement required to transport a hiker over a streambed, for example, highlights the pervasiveness of multijoint, multiplanar ground-based movement in the outdoors. It starts with a full-body push against the ground from the legs, then progresses through an integrated relay of pushes, moving from the ankles to the knees to the hips. Moreover, in the field this usually happens on one leg, and thanks to uneven terrain, usually off center or even sideways in direction. A standing arm push needed to push a car out of a snowdrift requires not only the basic large movers of the upper body (chest, shoulders, and arms), but the many smaller muscles in the core and peripheral areas that support your joints and correct sudden imbalances when your boots slide out from under you on the slush.

Real-world movements are also often conducted in more than one plane of movement. You may push a machine press in a path that is not allowed to veer from true north, but step outside to lift something heavy and it will be wobbling back and forth, here and there, and side to side as well. Most work in the gym has you working in a front-to-back plane of movement, but stabilizing your legs in a chimney on a climb requires lateral (or side-to-side) pushing strength, and a kayak stroke requires rotational pulling strength. Most important, all ground-based movements in the outdoors require a strong splint of muscle in the midsection to transfer forces between your upper and lower body, lest all your pulling, pushing, and rotating fold back against you like a noodle.

QUESTIONS, QUESTIONS

With bodybuilding and weight loss acting as such poor substitutes for the ordinary labor cut from our lives, it is little wonder we have lost touch with many of our instincts about physical work, and end up deferring so many decisions about how to become strong to outside experts. I once got a taste of our national befuddlement about the ways of fitness during a stint spent answering training questions online. *Outside* magazine put a point of entry on its web site a few years back where readers could send in their fitness questions to be answered by yours truly. I was going to be Izzy Mandelbaum, or at least the scribe who would field one or two questions out of a hundred or so every month, then call up the right expert and try to render the advice in plain language.

Some of the writers asked questions that seemed simultaneously simple and requiring of a PhD in biomechanics: "Should I do crunches or full sit-ups and why?" wrote one reader. I wanted to answer, but then I remembered how I once had asked this seemingly simple question of a sports-medicine physician, and he told me it was sort of too complicated to get into at the time. (Full sit-ups, in which the work is transferred from the abdominals to the hip muscles, can put stresses on your back, he said, even though that never stopped my grade school phys ed teacher from having us do full sit-ups.) "How much of your body weight do you push up when you do a push-up?" wrote another curious reader. I have always wanted to know the answer myself, actually. Surely it is out there somewhere, a phone call away. But I couldn't get past the larger question of how the answer would change anything about how to work out.

Some questions personified the very smartest sort of use of a would-be training expert. "I am 20 and snowboard constantly in the winter and spring," wrote a sensible girl from Maine named Mary. "Living on the east coast, I am often going through the park and hitting jumps with hard landings. What type of exercises can I do to help protect my knees against the abuse they take while I am snowboarding?" Talk about a sensible question. How come she is so proactive and rational at just 20, I thought to myself, when I just bounded out to learn to ski at 30 on legs like twigs?

For every question like this, though, there was one that made me wonder if training hasn't made us overly inhibited, or at least removed from our gut instincts about movement. "Is it harmful to combine weights and cardio exercise in the same workout?" wrote a reader from India. (India! This Internet thing is really something.) He said he lifted weights and then ran slowly for 40 minutes afterward, all of which would seem to resemble a day in the field followed by a brisk journey home. Or this: "I am a female who wants to work out my chest area to make it more firm. Will a few push-ups help, or do I need to bench press?" I wanted to say my hunch was that they are sort of the same, depending on some very minor technicalities that I was too undisciplined to investigate, so why not just do that which is the most fun?

The questions that gave me the most pause, however, were those where the workout I had recently provided, an attempt to merge the more resilient training maxims of the training literature into one five-month plan entitled the Shape of Your Life, left the reader in need of more follow-up: Why did our plan just tell you to run an hour every day during the endurance phase, when most workouts said differently? (Answer: I wanted to keep it simple. But maybe it's because I am a simpleton.) How were you supposed to merge sport-specific training in days toward the end of the month? (Answer: Neglecting to provide this information might have been an oversight.) What if I have not been able to improve my markers of endurance with the workout? (Answer: Maybe it is too easy for you.) How long should I rest between sets? My heart rate climbs precipitously, should it? How can I cycle through this workout again?

Once I calmed down from the feeling that I had written something simultaneously popular and confusing, I wanted to tell them all this: You all know how to work your muscles instinctively. You are created to do work, work that falls into a surprisingly small number of categories given the abundance of gear cluttering a gym floor. As core training innovator Paul Chek has written, to make it through the Darwinian maze, your body needed to push, pull, bend, rotate, squat, and step. Outside the gym, the six or so basic movements of human biomechanics all come naturally. If you had to move a pile of something heavy and were at all alert about the task at hand, chances are you would likely adopt good form. You would square your shoulders with the mass, flex your knees, breathe deeply, gird your core, pare down your movements in complexity, and work within the limits of your strength with control and success. Toddlers drop into deep squats to do the simplest things—and with no training at all. But we get to the gym and become confused. We curl dumbbells two inches, pull barbells behind our heads, and perfect the infinitesimally small bending of our knees on stair machines.

THE BENEFITS OF TRAINING

Here is the good news: If the typical training M.O. is superficial, your body is multidimensional and deep. It has the potential to express multiple athletic modalities—widely undeveloped skills ranging from easy endurance to explosiveness, from multidirectional speed to unassisted flexibility. In other words, you wouldn't know it

from the row upon row of elliptical trainers substituting themselves for fun, but vast and unlimited are the metabolic questions most of us have yet to ask of our muscles and tendons, capillaries, mitochondria, and neurons.

Should the American fitness dichotomy of body-shaping/athletic perfection leave you uninspired, this book is meant for you. There are better ways to work out and there are better reasons to work out than just looking good or winning races. There is a lengthy list of benefits to working out that have nothing to do with your appearance or competitiveness. Training can help with weight management, build a stronger heart capable of a lower resting heart rate, offset a decline in bone density, and help reduce excessive levels of body fat, which is not just a drag on your biomechanical efficiency but also a biologically active agent with inflammatory properties all its own. (Note: The deleterious effects of body fat mentioned here refer to levels in excessive amounts only. Nothing about this point should be taken to give comfort to those fat-eschewing athletes hiding their phobias behind a cover of training. You know who you are. You guys need to lighten up. Eat some ice cream.) The not-so-widely discussed benefits of training don't stop there: Both cardiac and strength training have been found to slow the neural degeneration of aging, have an anti-inflammatory effect within your blood vessels, reverse the premature muscle loss caused by working in a chairbound society, give you more energy, help combat stress, and cause the body to release human growth hormone, conferring a longevity and anti-aging benefit. For those wishing to live an adventurous life, training can allow you to challenge yourself physically without risking sports injury or the demoralization of limbs that quit before your will fades or ski pass expires. Training can make you the one the group selects when there's a log in the middle of the trail that needs to be moved, or when someone is needed to restock the woodpile for the nice people who loaned you their cabin. Training can boost your perception of your competence, which in turn will help broaden the range of experiences you take up in life.

ABOUT THIS BOOK

In the pages that follow you will find out why your body moves, both biologically and physiologically and this will help give meaning to how you train to make it move longer, with more force, power, flexibility, balance, and agility. It might also give you something to curl up with when the snow is piled outside and there's nothing worth watching on TV. You will learn the basic rules of training for endurance (Chapter 2), strength (Chapter 3), flexibility (Chapter 4), speed and power (Chapter 5), agility (Chapter 6), and balance (Chapter 7). You will learn how to add a dimension of sport-specific training to your workouts (Chapter 8). You will come across a guide to how you might integrate the disparate modalities of fitness training into one six-month calendar, to be recycled and reinvented year in and year out. (Chapter 9). Should you like the option and have the time, by all means give the training plan a try. But should your needs differ, plan on improvising, especially should the advice become too easy, too advanced, too tedious, too confusing, or too shocka-locka-ding-dong.

You will learn about nutrition—what you put in your body, and how that relates to weight management, health, and sports performance (Chapter 10). You will learn about some factors that help make you more resilient in coming back to a training plan when you falter (Chapter 11). That you *will* fall off the training wagon, again and again throughout your life, is the only fact in all of this of which there is any certainty.

You will be offered 50 basic principles that empower you to improvise with any of this advice (Chapter 12). A few unsponsored thoughts on gear are sprinkled in along the way.

This guide is meant for the broad cross section of readers not necessarily needing to drop multiple pant sizes but hoping instead for more purposeful and functional uses in the time they spend at the gym. In organizing the book, exercise descriptions and illustrations were placed in subject chapters and then cross-referenced alongside the final training plan in Chapter 9. To train at home, invest in dumbbells, a stability ball, and a yoga mat. A heart rate monitor is helpful but not necessary.

If there is one overall hope for this book, it is to invite the *Outside* reader to think about training less as a skill with gym equipment and more as skill with differing ideas about how the body changes. Think of the following pages as a guide to the better ideas about athleticism, a complement to hands-on help from trainers and coaches (because words and pictures can tell you only so much), a framework to help you evaluate ideas about training as they come along in the future, and most of all, a foundation for living an evolving, self-directed, and active life in the outdoors.

chapter 1

FEAR NOT THE TRAINING PLAN

FACE IT, TRAINING PLANS GIVE YOU A HEADACHE. If there's one thing that makes the normal person groan about the possibility of training, it is the sight of all those graphically enhanced instructions about **WHAT TO DO** in the gym and when, in how

many configurations and for how long, for how many weeks and at what percentage of your one-repetition maximum, all before reformatting the entire prescription to fit the next phase of some multimonth, stagger-tiered trajectory toward diabolically master-planned greatness. When all you really wanted to do was to firm up the old be-hind.

No matter how inspiring, well-designed, or colorful, every training book eventually arrives at a point where it dutifully crams its advice into orderly grids, workout homework purportedly to be carried out by you in the coming weeks and months. Some people like nothing more than an orderly plan laid out before them, a recipe that they can clip to a gym bag and check off each day as they pull on their running socks. But others see in these plans workouts meant only for the bionic man, Lance Armstrong, or some Brezhnev-era, Eastern-Bloc Olympic prospect. In their defense, most training plans do sort of threaten to squeeze all the fun out of it.

Before you read any further, then, it would be helpful to prepare you for any hesitation you may be experiencing about getting into a training plan, and why overcoming it can be a good thing.

Having an aversion to workout regimentation is probably far more widespread than any of the legions of fitness evangel-

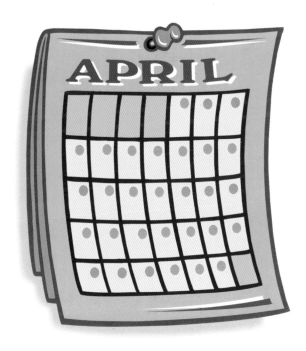

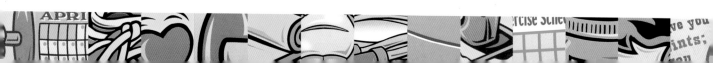

ists out there realize. In the rush to appear positive, upbeat, and basic good role models for the virtue of regular calisthenics, training plans often forget that for most of us, life is busy and serious enough as it is, all of which makes exercise a mostly unnecessary, moderately goofy business. What is working out, really, but a nondestructive escape from the daily grind: You run, you jump, you move things that are heavy, you try to see what it feels like to make your lungs burn and your muscles sore. It's good for you, but it's goofing around. In fact, you could say that training time is the least official, most unrestricted portion of our lives. But you wouldn't know that by the daunting tone and aching specificity of most training charts—what with their military-style abbreviations and triweekly obligations nestled into convenient multiweek blocks. Nor would you know, by their often omniscient tone, that many one-month training subunits are surely plotted around the schedules of magazine publishing more than some iron law of anatomical transformation.

INTUITIVE TRAINING IS OK, TOO

You don't have to organize your training across the entire year if you don't want to. Just by showing up, working a representative assortment of exercises, gradually progressing from controlling your body weight to external loads, balancing all the pushing with enough pulling, moving over a course of months from high numbers of easy repetitions to lower numbers of hard repetitions, and from long, slow, distance runs to shorter bursts at a greater intensity—will cause your body to undergo systematic improvement in its athletic performance

with no lengthy training handbook to show for it, especially if you are fairly new to this training business. (It's those with much less to improve about their anatomy who have to calibrate their training most carefully to achieve an effect.)

You see, in spite of how authoritative the fitness literature may appear, telling someone how to train is ultimately an educated guess. Some coaches and trainers surely have individual experience to draw on; the research on the ways of scheduling workouts is certainly extensive, and researchers have done much to chart the effects of changing training variables over the course of days, weeks, and months. But most would agree that designing workouts is more an art than a science. It is hard enough to do with any certainty for athletes getting ready for a specific goal at a specific time and place. For the rest of us, who merely wish to become more capable functionally or more well-rounded athletically, the application of one broad plan to the masses is by definition guesswork—the picking of choices from a menu of exercises. Like a chef, a trainer works with a fixed set of basic ingredients when writing up a plan, then fiddles with the combinations to get different results for different tastes. Most workouts follow the same four rules:

- A training plan needs enough individualization and specificity to be applicable to your goals and fitness level.

- A training plan needs enough progression to deliver results.

- A training plan needs enough recovery to permit improvement.

● A training plan needs enough variety to prevent boredom.

But once you do all that, what matters most is not so much the particulars of the plan, but *that* you train. Strangely enough, here is where a training plan can often provide its greatest asset.

FIVE GOOD REASONS FOR FOLLOWING A PLAN

A training plan may look like a numerical guide to how you exercise, but in reality its function is often more one of organizing behavior. Here are some ways that can happen.

Motivation. For the great majority of recreational athletes who are merely trying to work upward rather than to shave milliseconds—that would be you and me—much of the value of a plan is the discipline it offers, and much of the work of those who write them is more inspirational than educational. As a purely motivational tool, a training plan has no substitute: drafting a big-picture look at your year, giving yourself a concrete and variegated set of directions to follow month after month can fill in for the many, many reasons we can find not to work out.

Confidence. Following a systematic plan can boost your confidence in taking the step to enter a race or competition. You could just expand your runs every day when the mood strikes you, but wouldn't you rather place your trust in principles rather than your daily impulses? Should you wish to show up for an event and know that you are prepared to succeed, there can be no greater comfort than knowing you followed a plan to get there.

Simplicity. A calendar can make your training time involve less guesswork each day, including the guesswork as to whether or not you have done too much or too little. Over time, a lot of athletes lose their ability to recognize when they need a break. Organizing your training complete with recovery days will reduce your chances of slipping into the sort of endless training grind that stunts progress. It will also free your mind to focus on what you are doing, and not when, why, and how.

Progress. A long-range plan offers you insight on your progress. If you pause early in an endurance schedule to take note of, say, your 1-mile time at a given personal effort level, then take the same test after two months of training, you can see if your workout is challenging enough to move you forward. Because running progress especially is made in yearly increments more than monthly steps, a plan also gives you more of a baseline to use when drawing up next year's plan.

Organization. Finally, a plan is systematic. Just as you would rather not spend your money day in and day out for the rest of your life without some sort of organized financial objectives (or at least my wife would rather I not do so), when you organize how you exercise, you cycle through different periods of effort. This protects you from doing the same work endlessly, getting bored, and giving up.

FITNESS IS FOREVER

For the purposes of this book, the following material will compile a template that you can use to cycle your training toward goals, in this case, those of regular, biannual periods of peak fitness. What you do with these periods of peak fitness is yours to decide, of course. Some may wish to use them for skiing, others for cycling, and still others for climbing. Indeed, the broad variety of goals out there and the widely disparate training objectives required to get ready for, say, a paddling expedition versus a trail-hiking adventure will combine to mean that the singular plan contained in the coming chapters can do only so much. While this book will teach you the rough outline of how to tailor a training plan for a particular event, there are lots of great books out there to help you move toward a specific goal, such as a marathon, triathlon, or 10K. But chances are, just getting yourself to a point where you could confidently exert yourself in all modalities of fitness will mean you are in incredible shape.

PUTTING AN ADVENTURE ON THE CALENDAR

Most training books are written for coaches who must get athletes in shape for events on the horizon. This, of course, has little connection to how life works once you leave school and turn in your equipment. Most of us are no longer involved in predetermined athletic calendars, which means that if we want to get the benefits of training in an organized way, we have to find our own ways to structure our year. We have to be proactive.

One way to give structure and purpose to your training year is to pick out some ironclad, time-sensitive reason to get better—a trip somewhere beautiful and remote that requires a bag of gear and costs a lot of money and heartache if you show up out of shape—then buy the plane ticket and pay the registration fee months in advance to commit your attendance.

If you can swing the sometimes hefty fees, most adventure-travel companies offer paddling, cycling, trekking, and multisport vacations in exotic locales year-round. If you've never had the pleasure, active vacations are extremely habit-forming, simply because the food tastes better when you've pushed yourself during the day, the sightseeing is better when you are out in the elements, and the company is nicer when you have all been through some exhausting travail together. Better yet, if you excel at organizing travel, you can always choose to book your own cycling, paddling, or trekking vacations and forego the extra expense of doing it through a service. All of this would not only help make you more confident physically, but also an administrator of your own fun. We schedule events months in advance for other priorities in life, and there's no reason we can't do the same with training.

A SINGLE PLAN

While different sports carry different training objectives, there is much that links them, and the advice contained within these pages will shoot for the sweet spot in the broad middle between specificity and generality. It assumes your goal is to become broadly fit—armed with the endurance to run for an hour at 80 percent of your aerobic potential, with the strength to pull and push and squat your body for sets that number a dozen repetitions, the flexibility to fold effortlessly like a swan, the balance to stand on one leg, and the agility to skip rope like Evander Holyfield. More important, it assumes your goal is to know how to reinvent your own workouts throughout the years ahead, with different emphases as your goals change. With the realization that fitness is a lifetime change to be made in all of us, getting yourself into and out of regular fitness training cycles can be nothing less than a veritable insurance policy for sustainable training with a purpose.

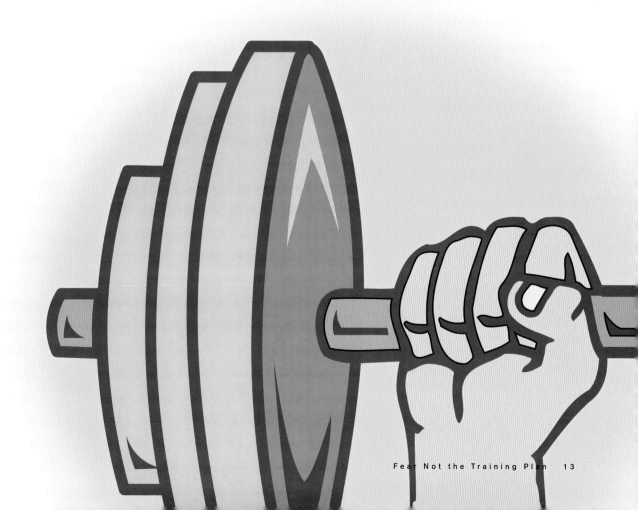

chapter 2

ENDURANCE

A word on how *NOT* TO THINK ABOUT RUNNING. They deserve better, but it's easy to dislike runners anyway. I trace my regretful PERIODS OF ANTI-RUNNERISM back to a perfectly agreeable and confident kid who took me out for a jog one crisp day

in the third year of the reign of Duran, Duran. I was 17 as I remember, and a pretty fit 17 year old. Would I go on a run? Sure, I said, pulling on my muscle shirt. I could knock off 50 push-ups. I had a pair of cut-offs and some Pumas. What's a run?

It turns out this guy was on the cross-country team, an after-school activity that at my high school tended to serve kids at risk for going on to college. We set out on a jog through our neighborhood, a jog that he shortly pushed faster, and after trying to stay with him until my lungs burned and my legs would slog no more I let him go. Maybe he let me go, actually. I'm still trying to put a better spin on that one. Watching him fade in the distance, the anxiety of failure washing over my brain like fog rolling into a harbor, I struggled with the realization that I could have probably whipped him in any number of contact sports, but he could just go. I ran sometimes, sure. But as a way to get to someplace, someplace where I could stop, put my hands on

my knees, and suck air until I no longer needed to puke. He was able to run for fun, as entertainment, like a person who reads books presumably reads books. In other words, he had endurance. To me that seemed more powerful than anything else you could say about a person, or at least me. So of course I hated him.

I drag you through this sorry tale of insecurity because I'm fully serious about the following half-baked point: The reason

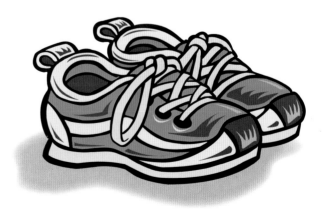

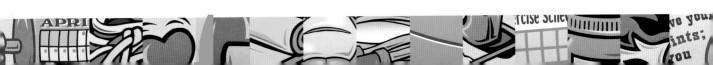

so many of us never try to build endurance is because of the way we tend to view people who have it. We think they're somehow more than human. It is the great painful secret we harbor when we say, "I think I will pick up running one of these days," while the mind quietly says ". . . and finally erase all doubt that I am not cut out to run." How else can they just do the same thing for mile upon mile? Either they are more disciplined, resilient, and endowed with lungs like an elephant, or long-distance athleticism is simply a test of boredom tolerance and they have brains like that of David Puddy, Elaine's dimwitted boyfriend on *Seinfeld* who once flew to India without so much as a paperback to keep him company.

ENDURANCE ENVY

Runners are different. They have a real skill, the Darwinian edge. On the day when we are all chased by men with long knives—a day that will surely come, mind you—the runners will outlast them. After the apocalypse, when all the cars are broken and the only medicine to save your child can be found in a village 20 miles down the road, the runners will get there, return before dinner, and need only a glass of cranberry juice and a copy of *Runner's World* to recover. They rule. Even if they don't see it that way. So we tend to think runners are better than we are, and because they don't really fight the image (probably more out of preoccupation with their hamstrings than egocentrism, in their defense), that keeps a lot of us—who doubt we're ever going to rule at anything—from running. This is wrong, because endurance is mostly a trick, and a trick that anyone can learn.

Here's the takeaway of this little endurance preamble: A lot of runners say they can't live without their run. Good for them. But don't try to be them. Most of us are never going to be people who don't feel like ourselves without a 5-mile run, and most of us wouldn't want to be. If you want to build your endurance, start thinking of running (or swimming or biking or rowing) as less of a lifestyle statement and more of a home repair project that may take a while, but with consistent attention, planning, and the usual periods of setback, will get done like anything else. The sooner people start thinking of a run as a purposeful piece of a larger project, the sooner they will quit hammering themselves for not being people who run just because they LOVE to run. Nobody loves to run. Not in the beginning anyway. And most runners don't think they are any better than you. They have other fish to fry. Shoes to buy, foot balm, that sort of thing. Who knows, develop a little endurance, and one day you may become someone who has developed a hard-to-shake habit of running, but that won't make you any better of a person. Just a person who runs when someone else does something else.

Endurance may seem like a triumph of the will, but in actuality it is a triumph of a metabolic efficiency. To build endurance is to expand your ability to use oxygen to keep your body moving. It results in being able to work longer, and eventually harder, and still feel comfortable.

Every one of us has an individual genetic ceiling to our ability to absorb oxygen. Like your ability to play a violin concerto at blazing speed and with precision, most of us are nowhere near close to our oxygen-sucking potential, which means that like those athletes who can go and go, what remains for you to do is to optimize yours. Easier said than done. Fortunately, there are but a few basic items of metabolic machinery that determine your oxygen-utilization potential, all of which respond to training.

BUILDING YOUR AEROBIC BASE

The key to the hoarding of oxygen comes down to making four basic improvements to the infrastructure of your limbs:

- Creating a deeper network of your so-called capillary beds—the spiderweb of threadlike vascular channels weaving themselves throughout your muscle and responsible for delivering freshly oxygenated blood to your muscle cells

- Stuffing your muscle cells with larger and more plentiful numbers of the intracellular bodies known as mitochondria—the engine rooms responsible for housing the aerobic burning of fats

- Raising your numbers of those certain oxidative enzymes necessary to turn the metabolic by-product known as lactate into fuel

- Causing more of your muscles, fast-twitch fibers, which tend to burn fuel quickly, to become converted to slow-twitch fibers, which tend to burn fuel slowly, thus making them capable of generating more aerobic energy

Like the repetitive work needed to build muscle and your heart, your capil-lary beds and mitochondria grow in number not through intensity, but through volume—through lengthy exposure to those somewhat easy-effort, so-called aerobic demands. The body can produce the fuel necessary to do work through three systems. All are working at some level at all times, but each has its own specialty. The aerobic energy system creates the fuel for movement (a compound known as ATP) through a lengthy process utilizing oxygen. The anaerobic energy system creates ATP more quickly, through a process that doesn't require oxygen, but which depletes itself of energy more quickly. The creatine-phosphate energy system creates ATP the quickest, and is depleted just as quickly as well. Each system takes the majority of the workload in different "windows" or intensity-defined segments of an extended effort. If you train too much above your aerobic window—meaning you train with too much intensity—you train your system to survive in a crisis environment, without developing more blood vessels and mitochondria. If you train too hard, too early, you also neglect the low-intensity muscular endurance work required to build up your tendons and other supporting muscles. You have to run for a long time to do both of those things, and that means running slow enough to be able to run long enough.

Training manuals refer to this sort of running as LSD, or long slow distance, and as the first leg of an endurance plan, it's a humble and patient exercise. (It may also be the reason so many runners are such stoic, loner types; you would think that it tends to draw in those willing to offer up their minds to hour upon hour of simmering sameness.) You simply have to put in the time at an easy but elevated pace to get these benefits. It is a requirement that would appear to render the acquisition of endurance less and less of a realistic possibility for those in a time-starved society such as ours. Increasingly, coaches are tailoring shorter workouts with high-intensity intervals early in a program. They do this to help runners build their VO_2 max (peak ventilatory volume) without offering up hours and hours to training. Others argue that running too slow delays teaching your legs the best biomechanics of swift running. But building an *aerobic base* through long, slow efforts at the beginning of a plan gives your body the best chance to acclimate to endurance, both metabolically and physiologically.

Building a long, slow, distance approach is also a method that makes acquiring endurance, at least at the amateur level anyway, enticingly democratic when compared to the genetic and financial litmus test required to become good at so many other gear-, geography-, and skill-based sports. There will always be a certain element of genetic potential at work in those at the highest level of endurance sports (favoring those born with greater numbers of the oxygen-hoarding slow-twitch muscle fibers). But at most levels, running just requires the right shoes, good basic biomechanics, and a lot of free time.

Even more enticing is the way that training for endurance has less to do with the number of miles you run than the amount of time you spend running. In developing an aerobic base, the body doesn't care how many miles you run, it cares about how long you were working and your intensity level. The level of a given effort for a set period of time is not only a far more meaningful yardstick for gauging endurance progress than that of distance, it is more democratic as well. Forty minutes at a 60 percent effort asks the same of *your* body that it asks of Lance Armstrong's. He merely gets much, much, much farther down the road than you do. If anything, amateur athletes often work harder in their frustrated, truncated, distance-focused efforts than do champion runners working things like closing speed and local muscular endurance.

As far as training advice goes, your body's three energy systems make intensity a more effective motivator than distance (how many miles you go), or pace (the time it takes you to go a certain distance). They also make the whole structuring of an endurance plan relatively simple. Your goal may be to one day run at a faster pace at a given heart rate—thus wringing more miles out of your minutes. You can even hope to one day work at higher heart rates for the same number of minutes. But to get to these goals, it helps to start out with a focus on time and effort alone. All of which means you can feel proud of even the slowest, most humble number of miles, provided you did them for the right duration and personal experience of intensity.

MEASURING INTENSITY

Over time, regular aerobic training has a way of making you intuitively sensitive to different levels of training intensity and how they affect your body. But in the beginning, you can gain more control over your efforts by learning how to gauge your effort level and target your training accordingly. You can do so with ascending degrees of precision, depending upon your goals and interest.

Ballpark Intensity:
Your Rate of Perceived Exertion

When it comes to training endurance there are three basic intensity zones—the moderate intensity of your aerobic energy pathway, the even easier intensity used to merely flush the system on an active rest day, and the harder effort used to push the upper limits of your aerobic energy system. The workout that this book (and nearly every other aerobic training plan) offers uses these three general zones to organize your training efforts (more on those later). But once you know this principle, how do you put it into action? Almost everyone has a watch to tell you how long you have been running, but trying to determine the slice of data that reflects your intensity is another story.

The easiest way is to guess, of course, basically asking yourself, "So, how hard does this feel, anyway"? This is known as your rate of perceived exertion, or RPE in training circles, and it basically means estimating how hard you are working on a scale of 1–10.

To use your RPE in a run, you might simply tell yourself to keep your effort level at say, a 6, in order to try to stay at a zone you could maintain for an hour. (You'd probably get the same result, however, just heading out on the road and telling yourself, I have to hold my pace for an hour, how fast should I go?) This may sound low-tech, but studies show that RPE scales tend to line up surprisingly close with "hard" measures of exertion that will be explained shortly. You don't have to invest in any fancy gear to keep your intensity level in check, with RPE, not as long as you trust yourself to deliver a realistic appraisal of how hard you are working, compared to how hard you could be working.

Heart-Rate Monitors

There are some obvious drawbacks to simply guessing your exertion level. Just as a lot of people say they watch only an hour of television a day, when asked to guess the intensity of their run, a lot of people will fudge the numbers. Others could underestimate how hard they are working; on some days the wind, hills, or dehydration can make your body work harder at a slower pace than you would expect. In psychology research, this is referred to as the limitations of self-report. You could take people's word for it, but then again, they might be in a bad mood or just not in touch with their body signals and be unable to gauge their effort. Here is where heart-rate monitors come into the picture. These units, which take a real-time reading of your heart rate every few seconds and transmit it to a watch for digital display, cost anywhere from $60–$300 and tell you how many beats your heart is clanking out in a minute. Basic versions can also give your average heart rate for a run, offer stopwatch functions, and allow you to program in little target zones that will chime when you get going too hard or too easy and wander out of your self-determined training zone. Higher-end monitors can offer a host of other functions, from how many calories you have supposedly burned off, to a projected estimate of the aerobic yardstick known as VO_2 max, to spitting your training log out into your computer to be gazed at wistfully while your family stands at the door, waiting for you to get off the computer and join them for an afternoon in the park. A great thing, no?

To outdoorsy purists, checking your watch to see what your heart is doing during your 40-minute trot must sound like a great way to spoil The Only Good Thing I Have All for Myself in My Entire Day, Especially Since We Got that Needy Lab Who Always Wants to Join Me. I was one of those. The idea of having to learn which number related to your running or swimming or cycling heart rate meant what in terms of your training goals seemed like purposefully adding some IRS form to your kid's paper-route earnings—an unnecessary encumbrance and distraction from the purity of stepping outside and running. But consider this: Aside from how to tell time, the primary thing you need to know in order to train endurance is how intensely your body is working, and your heart rate remains the most obvious measurement of effort. Why guess if you can watch and learn?

Besides giving you more confidence at lower heart rates, and permission to ease up at higher heart rates, an accurate heart-rate reading can triangulate subtle improvements in endurance you wouldn't appreciate otherwise, like being able to run your regular route at a lower average heart rate, and for longer. Sometimes it is this very proof of progress that helps you stick it out. In other words, heart monitors may look like some sort of gear fetish appealing only to die-hard accountants of their workouts, but it's the average person just learning about endurance who benefits the most from picking up a watch and strap.

Especially now that they cost little more than a decent pair of shoes.

ORGANIZING YOUR DATA

It's one thing to know your effort level, but its another thing to know what to do with those numbers. Take a minute to consider the big picture: Your resting heart rate, the rate it beats when you get out of bed in the morning, is about as low as it goes. Often it comes in at just less than 50 beats per minute. (Elite athletes have hearts so large and productive they don't see the need to beat more than 30 times per minute.) Your top-end heart rate on the other hand, is not what it used to be, no matter how well you are conditioned. Your maximum heart rate was at its highest with the teensy-weensy heart you were given at birth, when it could potentially, theoretically at least, bang out a zippity 220 beats per minute at its maximum. This high rate of speed is a by-product of diminutiveness. Listen to your dog's heart sometime, chances are it's really hammering.

During her visit to the ultrasound man, our embryonic child was ripping away at about 144 beats a minute. To move less blood per stroke and around a quicker circuit, a smaller heart has to beat far more frequently, even at rest. Each year your maximum heart rate decreases, however, first as your heart gets bigger, and then as you age into adulthood. Some of this is loss of potential based on genetic factors having nothing to do with fitness—like the actual size of your heart—and some has to do with age-related decline that also has little to do with fitness. By your 20s and 30s the fastest anyone's heart can possibly beat is somewhere in the range of 180 to

200 beats per minute, and by midlife that number dips as low as the 160s.

But here's the upshot: People can feel their eyes begin to glaze over when training advice turns to a discussion of numbers and percentages, but heart-rate monitoring is really all one big conversation about the same 60-odd number range. Given that people generally work out at half their maximum heart rate or higher (any lower and you are just another person unpacking the groceries), and given that people rarely get above 90 percent of their maximum, this whole bewildering notion of monitoring your heart takes place in a fairly tight window somewhere between the numbers 100 and 160. If you can keep track of your golf score, you can keep track of your optimal heart rate training zones.

Many believe that getting a maximum heart rate helps you for training according to four intensity zones: recovery zone, aerobic zone, threshold zone, and your anaerobic zone.

Your Recovery Zone

At roughly 30–60 percent of your maximum heart rate—anywhere between roughly 60 to 110 beats per minute for a person with a maximum heart rate of 187 like me—you can generally count on your body operating in an elevated but low-intensity zone useful for "recovery" runs. This entails activity of some sort that will increase your blood flow, albeit easy enough to not even approach the same area code as a hard run. Recovery zone efforts are meant not so much to condition you, as to speed the healing processes a day or so following a more taxing effort, by working at a heart rate that won't add any new

stressors into your sore system. You look pretty ridiculous running or cycling at such a slow pace, but you feel better faster and as a result are able to work harder on the days you work hard.

Your Aerobic Zone

Between 60–75 percent of your maximum heart rate—110 to 140 for me, to continue the example—your body is better able to absorb oxygen. This is because you are working hard enough to be aerobic (you are breathing harder than normal, basically), yet you are still working easy enough that your aerobic system is capable of doing the largest share of the workload.

Your Threshold Zone

Moving another notch up the effort scale, somewhere in the not-so-usefully vague parameters that are 75–85 percent of a person's best effort—140 to 160 beats per minute in my system, or a pace you could sustain for no more than an hour for those even at the top of their game—there lies a curious span in training time. Here is where we tend to see the so-called anaerobic threshold (AT), also referred to as the lactic threshold (LT) or simply threshold, the stage where your body starts to move from predominantly aerobic-fueled training into predominantly anaerobic-fueled training. Because here are the beginnings of exertion at a level high enough that your body has to over-rely on the anaerobic system to keep burning energy at this pace, and the anaerobic by-product known as lactic acid will begin piling up in your muscles faster than your aerobic system can absorb it, and the system has set in motion the wheels of its own shut-off mechanism. Contrary to popular belief, your "threshold" is less of a line in the sand than a gradual tipping of the scales, but it can be whittled down to a process that occurs within a fairly tight window of 5 or 6 degrees in your heart rate, nonetheless.

Provided you have put in enough time training aerobically to make the most of your oxygen, training in short bursts in the threshold zone, separated by short, slightly easier segments—*interval training*—can help your body learn to tolerate increased lactic acid, ultimately helping lengthen the duration at which your body can tolerate near-anaerobic efforts. By training just above and just below this threshold, you effectively cheat the system. Because the effort was punctuated with rests, it ends up putting you at threshold for longer than you could otherwise tolerate, all of which makes you stronger at the point where you once began to falter. Your body can tolerate only so much threshold training in a given training cycle before becoming worn out, which is why you don't do it endlessly, but rather cycle in and out of incorporating intervals from year to year.

Your Anaerobic Zone

Finally, to finish this discussion of training zones, working at anything higher than 85 percent of your maximum heart rate—the 160s and 170s on my heart-rate monitor—would be considered hard anaerobic runs for most of us, though elite runners can get into the low 90s of their maximum heart rate without passing their threshold. These are the kind of runs you see on *COPS*. They tend to last about as long, and end as badly. Training at 85 percent of your total heart rate potential or higher will increase the output of your anaerobic system. You can train here to build sprint speed, but it has little place

in an endurance training program. Do too much work above threshold and your body shifts more of its energy production over to getting fast, rather than long lasting.

Finding Your Maximum Heart Rate

In order to find three zones one must first determine the theoretical number that is your maximum heart rate, then apply the percentages for each zone. A popular low-tech method for finding your maximum heart rate has been to subtract your age from 220. If you were 20, that meant your heart could beat a maximum of 200 beats per minute, and by 40, according to this formula, your max heart rate was supposed to be no more than 180 beats per minute. However, this 220 minus age formula is a statistical average produced in a study, and can be an inaccurate yardstick. Variations on calculating MHR have emerged in recent years, such as multiplying your age by .85 and then subtracting the total from 217. Then there is the fact that your maximum heart rate varies from sport to sport, thanks to the physiology of blood flow. Leaning over your bike with blood moving to your legs, for instance, your heart rate just can't get as high as it can while running upright. When your torso is prone in a cold pool, your maximum heart rate is reduced even more. (Compared to your MHR for running, you need to subtract 3 beats per minute for rowing, 5 beats per minute for cycling, and 14 beats per minute for swimming.)

Once you consider the fact that you will never need to train at your maximum heart rate, and that the central organizing point for a training run is your threshold, finding a perfect number for your maximum heart rate is as questionable a goal as it is a fact.

ANAEROBIC THRESHOLD
(An Even Better Use of Your Heart-Rate Monitor)

Heart-rate training zones are a general approach to training within our three energy systems, but their limitations have come into view over the past few years. Does nature really design people of all fitness levels to be aerobic between a 60–75 percent effort? Smells a little fishy. Though training zones may provide a general yardstick for a large readership, people are surely more individual than these broad parameters suggest. The vagueness of training zones becomes especially pertinent as athletes become more highly trained, the location of these training zones relative to their maximum heart rate begins to rise, and their spans become smaller.

All of which begs the question: If your primary goal during a long, slow, distance run is to stay below your anaerobic threshold—a good 20 beats per minute below threshold if you want to be sure of putting in the time necessary to build oxygen utilization—and if this threshold is potentially narrower and a higher percentage of your maximum heart rate depending on your level of training; and if your maximum heart rate is such a potentially inaccurate guessing game in the first place; if all this is true, why figure out your maximum heart rate and the corresponding workload zones in the first place? Why not just figure out your anaerobic threshold?

It turns out that while your maximum heart rate and corresponding intensity zones derived from it are useful benchmarks, you can both simplify and better individualize your training by nailing down one simple number: the heart rate corresponding to your anaerobic threshold, which is a reliable principle, if not a precise point. There are a variety of ways trainers have come up with to identify subjectively when you have reached your anaerobic threshold. All are somewhat inexact. Here are several such ways to tell if you have reached your threshold. (All tests should be done when well rested, warm, and well hydrated.)

Your Breathing Gets All Messed Up

The simplest test of your threshold is a perceived exertion test. Set out on a run, gradually increase your speed every five minutes (you need to spend a few minutes at a given pace to let your systems establish their responses), and mark the eventual point where you notice a sudden change in your breathing. Once it becomes less controlled, you are at your anaerobic threshold heart rate. You should also have noticed your legs developing a burning feeling. Both effects are due to the accumulation of lactic acid at this heart rate. Your breath will be ragged, hard to control, and too strong to permit the back and forth of simple conversation. You don't have to be able to give a Shakespearean monologue, mind you, you just need to hold up your end of a conversation. Contrary to what you might think, you aren't suddenly breathing differently out of need for more oxygen, but because the extra presence of lactic acid in your blood has affected your brain's center for controlling your breath.

Your Rate of Breathing Is Tied to Your Footsteps

If you can breathe in over the course of three steps you are likely aerobic. If you are breathing in for only two steps, and then out for two steps, you are likely beginning to go anaerobic. By a one-breath-to-one-step ratio, chances are you are anaerobic at this heart rate.

Your Heart Rate Can't Keep Up with Your Effort Level

One of the oldest measures of your anaerobic threshold is known as the Conconi Point, named after an Italian cycling coach who used this method as early as 1982 to train champion racers. Conconi noticed that while the heart rate rises with increases in intensity, by a certain point you will notice that increasing your intensity doesn't cause the heart rate to jump quite as much. After warming up, increase your effort every five minutes, checking your heart rate. When your heart rate doesn't jump as high after an increase, you have found your anaerobic threshold.

Find Your Average Heart Rate for an Hour-Long Cycling Race, Then Subtract 10

Lance Armstrong's cycling coach Chris Carmichael has long advocated finding your anaerobic threshold pace via a test of your maximal sustainable pace, a healthy but restrained clip he refers to as your steady state. To find that, he recommends you find the average pace of your best effort over the span of an hour—otherwise known as your 10K pace—and subtract 10 beats a minute.

Find Your Average Heart Rate for a 30-Minute Running Race

Because you can generally cycle twice as long as you can run, to test your anaerobic threshold via running, you would take the average heart rate of your best effort over 30 min-utes, also loosely known as your 5K pace, because these are roughly 3-mile efforts. Some even say your average 20-minute race pace is a reasonable threshold heart rate.

Cycle Until You Can't Keep Up

Sit on a cycle ergometer, keep your cadence at a steady clip (90 RPMs is good), and gradually raise the resistance in three-minute increments until your legs can't hold the starting RPM.

AND FOR THE REALLY DETERMINED . . . BLOOD-LACTATE TESTING

Spend enough time pondering the many ways to guess whether your body has crossed its anaerobic threshold and you start to get hungry for the raw data. Believe it or not, that's easier than it looks. Your anaerobic threshold is a relatively fixed point in your heart rate where your muscles can no longer absorb the by-product known as lactic acid, or *blood lactate*. If you want to get to the bottom of exactly where your body begins to accumulate lactic acid, and if you want to invest a few hundred bucks in some jock-lab gear about the size of an iPod, you always have the option of cutting to the gold standard of intensity measurement—which is to stop mid-run, prick your finger, dab it in a lactic acid measuring device, and actually test the millimoles of lactic acid per liter present in your blood. It may involve blood and Kleenexes, but this sort of test is the surest way around all those heart-rate training zones, calculating your maximum heart rate, guessing your level of perceived exertion, or testing any of the ways to estimate your lactate threshold. That's because while all the above tests make subjective judgments about your body's energy system transition, this one is the real thing, completely individualized to your body in the shape it is in right now, doing the work you are doing right now.

By the time you're taking samples of your blood, of course, you are no longer a casual participant in all of this endurance cosmology. Apparently it used to freak out the Americans when they looked over and saw the Eastern Bloc athletes drawing blood samples during Olympic competition trial warm-ups 30 years ago. Today, however, blood-lactate testing has become an option for the highly curious amateur as well as the highly funded elite, and could very well present the final frontier of smart endurance training. Not only does blood-lactate testing cut through all the guesswork of conventional heart-rate training, it is also increasingly affordable and portable. Blood-lactate analyzers now run in the high $300 range and can fit in your seat bag or fanny pack—should you possess the self-assuredness to wear such a thing. Few trainers outside the uppermost echelons of training seem to know about blood-lactate testing, however, and getting your hands on one isn't easy. You can buy a heart-rate monitor in any mall for instance, but finding a portable blood-lactate analyzer usually means researching the products on the Internet.

I did this, and one proprietor, a former Swiss ski coach operating a distributorship in Canada, sent me Lactate Pro, a unit the size of a small music player. It showed up in a small bag containing three essential components: a small handheld display, a skin-pricking device of the sort used by diabetics to check their insulin, replaceable sharps, and several long chains of individually sealed test strips. You insert the strips halfway into a slot in the unit, prick yourself, dab the exposed tip of the other end of the strip into the drop of blood oozing from your fingertip and wait for the machine to show your blood-lactate level. Seeming simultaneously simple and daunting—especially the thought of producing blood on purpose—when mine arrived I put it in my drawer and decided not to look at it for a month.

Many believe your blood lactate reaches its threshold at a universally specific volume, specifically, that of 4 millimoles (m/mol) per liter of blood. But even this assumption—one currently making the rounds at the highest-level exercise science conferences—is flawed. Some athletes do indeed reach their anaerobic threshold at 4 m/mol blood lactate per liter of blood, but many other highly trained athletes do not do so until 8 or even 12 m/mol per liter. Like everything else in training, it turns out the 4 m/mol figure is merely an average, and one based in this case on a single study of 16 subjects 25 years ago. What this means in practical terms is that should you actually get your hands on a blood-lactate measurement device, then go to the trouble of running yourself ragged and watching your heart rate climb before pricking your finger, merely trying to tie a heart-rate effort to a point where your monitor reads 4 m/mol blood-lactate level isn't enough. You have to find out the specific blood-lactate level at which *your* body ceases to keep up with reabsorbing lactic acid, and determine the heart rate at which you reach that level.

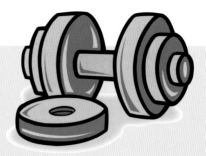

IRONMAN DeBOOM

Tim DeBoom won the Ironman Triathlon twice in a row, but after interviewing him once I was pleasantly surprised to learn how he too has to think about some of the same ordinary numbers I wrestle with at my gym. The specifics: His maximum heart rate is in 180–190 range. He thinks his threshold currently falls in the 160s or high 170s, and when I spoke with him in the off-season, he was spending all his time in one-to two-hour long, slow, distance training, running at intensities far below—140 to 155 beats per minute—the high end of his aerobic level. Boring, you say?

Because his body uses oxygen so well, DeBoom can keep that easy heart rate while tearing down the road at just over a six-minute-mile pace, and can do so for the duration of your typical feature length film. The reason DeBoom can "jog" faster than you and I can sprint is due to four primary factors: his biomechanical efficiency; his having a metabolic infrastructure composed of far more extensive capillary beds; his higher overall numbers of the intracellular oxygen-processing engine rooms known as mitochondria; and his greater numbers of those key enzymes and transporters that help redirect lactic acid out of the muscle cell and into the body's fuel-processing pathways. He got those from gradually seeing improvements with each passing year, rather than month. "It takes your body a long time to build up to a fast marathon," he says. "It took me eight or nine years, because I didn't have a running background. It's taken me years to get to the level where I can train three sports a day, 30 hours a week," he says. "I don't recommend it for everyone." Moreover, when DeBoom does finally get to the four weeks toward the end of his base-building period—he spends his time running short bursts above and below his threshold heart rate. Lest you think your job is to do these for an hour or even 20 minutes, even the longest an Ironman like DeBoom will run at threshold is the length of a few songs on a CD, maybe 6–10 minutes. "By now I know my threshold by feel," says DeBoom, who estimates his lactic acid starts to accumulate around the high 160s. "You want to train above it and then below it, but that's where you want to race at."

According to endurance coach Juerk Feldman, one way to find your individual anaerobic threshold through blood-lactate testing goes like this:

1. Run yourself, gradually, to a hard pace. Run 6 minutes easy, then 6 minutes medium, and then 6 minutes hard.

2. Stop and measure your blood-lactate level, as you should at this point have crossed your anaerobic threshold.

3. Drop to a pace that lets you run 40 beats per minute slower, and hold it for 5 minutes. Measure your blood-lactate level, raise your pace by 5 beats per minute for 5 minutes, and repeat. Repeat until your reading stops getting smaller and starts getting bigger; that is the heart rate where your body becomes anaerobic.

I completed this gold standard test of my lactate threshold heart rate and it told me something very specific and very useful for future training runs: I reached my lactate threshold at 150 beats per minute. What that means, according to my very blood, is that I should be running long, slow, distance runs in the 130s and 140s (20 beats or so less than threshold), and that I should be doing interval runs at a pace just over and just under 150 beats per minute. This was right about where the heart-rate training zones had predicted I should do these things, which should be comforting to those who choose to test their thresholds through low-tech methods. But it also was indisputable, which was inspiring in a way that merely listening to your breathing would never be able to duplicate. If I wanted to increase my endurance, I now had an ironclad standard to pass.

EVERYONE'S SHOOTING FOR THE SAME BASIC NUMBERS

Lest all this talk about numbers make you groan, keep in mind that you're not alone when venturing into the sometimes-baffling mathematics game of endurance training. Everyone, even the very best athletes out there, is trying to figure out where his or her body's energy systems fall within these same numbers.

In many ways, we will never be Tim DeBoom, of course, which makes all of this comparison-making a little, well, presumptuous. But if you can see the relative similarities between his training at 160-beat intervals with your interval training at 150- beat intervals, the fact that he's running nearly twice the speed that you are seems less discouraging, the intensities you share more inspiring, and the pace you are running, utterly meaningful.

THE ESSENTIALS OF ENDURANCE TRAINING

Given all that we have learned here then, because it is surely a lot to keep track of in trying to get so you can swim or cycle for the length of a couple of sitcoms, it would be nice to have it all boiled down to a couple of easy maxims. With that in mind, if you only remember 10 things about endurance, let them be these:

1. Learn your numbers. Learn your anaerobic threshold heart rate in beats per minute, and then subtract 20 or so beats to get a mid-range idea of your

aerobic heart rate. Forget about finding your maximum heart rate, and forget about how many miles you are running. Keep your focus on these two mileposts of intensity, and, to help you get a yardstick on days you leave your monitor at home, the pace you take them at in minutes per mile.

2. Begin by running at a pace where you can carry on a conversation.

3. Gradually increase your frequency until you are running, swimming, or cycling four to five days a week.

4. Every other week increase your duration by roughly 10 percent.

5. Gradually build your duration until you reach 60–90 minutes a day for runners, and if you can spare it, two or more hours a day for cyclists.

6. If you can, do #5 for 4 months.

7. Then, try to get 4–6 weeks of twice-weekly interval training. After testing to find your lactate threshold, structure multiple sets of brief runs above and below this heart-rate intensity, beginning with those intervals below your threshold rate double the length of those intervals above your threshold rate.

8. Increase your interval lengths until they reach 10 minutes in length.

9. Gradually shorten your recovery periods until they equal half your interval lengths.

10. If you are really interested in seeing the numbers behind the results, twice a month, head to the track to gauge your performance. Run a mile at speeds that used to make your heart race, and you'll know you have a bigger engine. You will also have more than a running routine; you will have endurance.

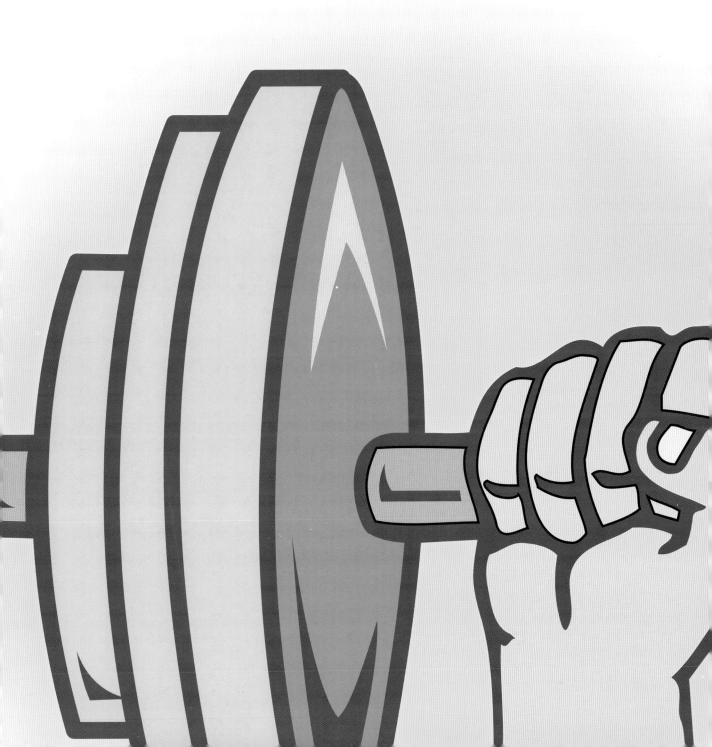

chapter 3
STRENGTH

AT ANY GIVEN TIME you can walk into a state-of-the-art health club, take in **THE STATE-OF-THE-ART** equipment, and watch a room full of bright and capable people doing things that **DON'T ESPECIALLY RESEMBLE, WELL, STRENGTH.**

Strength is the force needed to move a certain level of resistance for a set amount of distance, usually the range of motion of your arms or legs. Strength also describes the muscular endurance necessary to move that resistance for a certain number of times before tiring. But the gym is another thing. Over there is a compressed-looking guy banging out a batch of one-armed bicep curls. His bicep isn't able to take his dumbbell through a full extension of his arm, however, so he's short-arming it, turning a joint that's supposed to sweep as broad as a windshield wiper into one that ticks like a metronome set on rave. He's getting strong, but at a movement spanning the length of a pickle.

Ten feet in the other direction another would-be strongman is experiencing the charms of a lat pull-down machine. That's the contraption where you pull weighted plates up a guided track by tugging downward on a horizontal bar. There's basically only one instruction on the lat pull-down—

pull the bar to your chest. Our man is pulling it to the back of his neck. When in life outside the gym will you ever need to pull something behind your neck? Over at the squat rack, a different man strengthens the muscles of his hips and legs, sort of. Squats are those lifts where you either

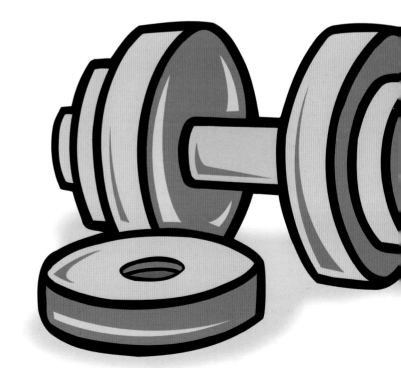

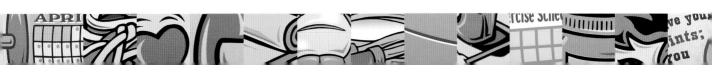

hold dumbbells at your side or rest a barbell on the back of your neck, dip your rear to an altitude just above chair level, then stand back up. In order to squat a whole lot of weight, our man is squatting just to the height of a bar stool.

A common thread runs through these flawed improvisations—doing things in the weight room that have little connection to the way your body works in the real world. The reason for all this fevered activity is because strength training has undergone a veritable renaissance in the past 20 years. Once the domain of bodybuilders and fitness zealots, it was only relatively recently that certain changes came along to usher the masses into weight rooms, to the point where lifting weights is now the most popular sport in the country. Surely one of the most obvious reason lifting weights has become so popular has to do with the way our ideal bodily form seems to be getting more hypertrophied while the actual form of most Americans deteriorates.

STRENGTHENING MOVEMENTS, NOT MUSCLES

Strength is a more sustainable goal when you detach it from thinking about body parts and think instead about movements. As stated earlier, biomechanically speaking, we do six basic things: push, pull, bend, rotate (or throw), squat, and step (and stepping and squatting are almost the same thing). We can push, pull, and step in three separate planes of movement, from the upper body, lower body, while anchored on firm ground, or on an unstable surface. But that's about it. Six basic movements. We can do an innumerable number of activities in the execution of those six primary movements, but they still come down to some variation of pushing or pulling, bending, stepping, and squatting.

But you don't learn these sorts of multijoint, multiplanar movements on most strength machines, those pin-loaded devices that clutter the health club floor, or even most bench-based lifts. Gym routines tend to work only one muscle at a time, are limited to one plane of movement, and are often buttressed or supported by padding, especially around the back and core. To their credit, strength machines tend to be idiot-proof. You don't have to lift plates, which means you don't have to risk dropping them on your foot, and you can only do exactly one thing on a strength machine, which is exactly what the machine allows. Strength machines, as we said earlier, will isolate muscles to an even greater extent than traditional weight lifting. Where the free-weight version of the bench press requires using your shoulders to stabilize the weight laterally, the machine version of a bench press asks only that you push the weight away from your chest. As such, strength machines are useful introductions to strength development for the highly deconditioned as well as those trying to do the extremely limited efforts needed to rehabilitate an injured joint or limb. While newer, so-called ground-based cable machines are beginning to make machine training more functional, most traditional strength machines share a similar set of liabilities. You sit. You push weights in a factory-set plane of movement. You do so with two hands supporting one another, (and hiding the fact that your one side is probably weaker than the other side) and you do so while cradling those pesky support muscles with back, leg, and arm rests.

An emerging body of research into "functional training" now identifies these as faulty assumptions about how we become strong. Once out of the gym we do very little that requires strength while sitting. Not only does sitting while lifting remove your core stabilizing muscles from a task, but by keeping the weights confined to a predetermined track, and isolating, or removing all work from the small stabilizing muscles supporting a movement, machines build strength that has little transferability to strength as it is required in the real world.

THE MYSTERY OF GAINING GYM STRENGTH THAT TRANSFERS TO THE FIELD

To gain useable strength, you have to design a workout around an idea known as the *transfer of training*, or whether what you do transfers into added capacity for work in the real world. While functional trainers have regularly claimed transferable strength is that which is multijoint, multiplanar, and unstable, researchers have broken the subject down even further. For strength to transfer from the gym to the field, some now say your gym exercises must be comparable to what you do in the field according to four factors: speed, range of motion, type of contraction, be it a shortening, lengthening, or enduring force, and the overall sequence of muscles involved in a contraction.

In other words, the speed with which you overcame resistance in the gym, be it fast or slow, will determine if you can do the same in the field (hence the benefit of periodic fast lifting, otherwise known as power training). For your work to pay off, the range of motion, be it wide or narrow, must also be comparable to the range of motion you will need to lift something in the field (hence the need for curls and squats that extend deeper than just inches). The type of muscular contraction with which you lifted a weight in the gym, whether shortening (also known as concentric), lengthening (also known as eccentric), or enduring (also known as isometric and isotonic), must be comparable to the type of contraction your strength will be manifested in outdoors (hence the need for control with the weight you are using during the pushing, lowering, and holding stage of a lift). Finally, to transfer into real-world use, your strength must be executed in a sequence of movements likely to be replicated outdoors (hence the need for multijoint movements—and utter lack of need for something like behind-the-neck lat pull-downs). Exercise researchers can fight over the nuances of these distinctions, but for most people gearing up for outdoor sports, once you have built a basic level of bodily strength through traditional weight training, getting strong boils down to the following:

- Strength is manifested in movements.

- Strength is manifested in the use of multiple joints in succession.

- Strength is manifested in three planes of movement in off-balance and upon unstable settings.

- Strength is manifested in different rates of force production or speed.

THE BASICS OF STRENGTH TRAINING:

It helps to take a minute to review exactly how most trainers advise a person to organize the beginning, middle, and end of a typical strength-training plan. Here are some of the basics.

Get Warm, Then Get Familiar

If you really want to develop new strength, you will need to first get warm through 10 minutes of brisk activity. Warm muscles move greater resistance than cold muscles. Budget this time in addition to the 45 minutes you'll need to work through a strength-training session. That will give you a generalized warm-up, but to acquaint your body with the specific movement that is to follow, you will also benefit from preceding every loaded exercise with an unloaded dry run. Such movement-specific warm-ups acclimate your body to the movement pattern through its fullest range of motion, which helps ensure that you will develop strength in the most functional manner possible.

Intensity Progression

At the start of any strength-development program, trainers will often advise you to put some time into building a foundation of basic strength. The idea of a strength foundation is vague, but it's generally believed that you ensure your greatest chance of success through: beginning with weights light enough that you can push them for multiple sets at 15–20 repetitions, building enough strength to control your own body weight for 15–20 push-ups, pull-ups, crunches, and controlled descents to a squat, and a half minute of your core stabilized in a side plank.

Should these requirements prove difficult, here is where modified body-weight exercises or traditional strength machines are more than appropriate. If you have a hard time with five push-ups, for instance, you can do a sitting machine press, or try push-ups from your knees or against the side of a table. If you have a hard time doing five chin-ups, as many people carrying extra weight have experienced, you can sit and pull down a weight less than that of your body on the stationary equipment or pull yourself up from beneath a picnic table or waist-high bar.

Once you can easily do 15–20 of the big four body-weight exercises—push-ups, pull-ups, crunches, and squats—they become less strength building and more muscular endurance exercises, meaning you are ready to move on from the over-supported domain of machine training to more advanced resistance training. Though for many, just reaching a point where you can control your body weight in multiple steps, squats, pushes, pulls, rotations, and extensions is all the strength you will ever need.

Reps

Reps, or the number of times you choose to move a resistance in a repetitive set, are really just a way to decide how much intensity you're going to put your muscles through. The higher the reps, the lower the intensity—you simply can't move something at the high end of your strength limits a whole lot of times. Using high reps in the beginning keeps your weight modest. Using lower reps later on signals a move toward more intense, shorter durations with a given resistance. Much research has gone into how different ranges of reps affect your muscles differently.

For the first portion of any strength-training plan, researchers recommend using weights light enough that you can do every lift in multiple sets of 15–20 repetitions. For those seeking greater strength and muscular size, trainers recommend lifting enough weight for 10–12 repetitions. According to biomechanical principles, a weight that you can lift only 10–12 times is 70–75 percent of your one-rep maximum (1RM), or the heaviest weight you could ever lift just once. Unless you are training for weight-lifting competition, actually lifting your one-rep maximum is something you have little need to experience; doing your hardest lift possible is strictly for show, and it's not especially safe and not much of a show at that. Practically, lifting your max has little value as well, as the output of a one-off for any lift is too low to build strength.

But it helps to think of a 10–12 rep set in relation to your total strength potential, because it underscores the fact that you will actually get stronger over time. It works like this: When a 10–12 rep resistance becomes too easy—when you feel like you have perhaps two or three more reps in you, for two workouts in a row—you know for a fact that the weight is no longer an overload and that you will see little gain in strength until you increase the resistance. Anything lighter than the resistance you can move 10–12 repetitions and you will be building local muscular endurance, as opposed to strength. Anything heavier than the resistance you can move 10–12 repetitions and you will be building muscular size more than strength.

Pay even more attention to how each set ends; it should not be too easy to get that tenth, eleventh, or twelfth repetition up. While many strength trainers advocate lifting to whatever repetition it is that diminishes good form, others say lift until your limbs actually fail. Some bodybuilders even try lifting to failure plus one or two more, which would seem to occur after an extra moment's rest with the weights still in your hand. But the downside of training to failure, or training to failure plus two for that matter, is more apparent when considering what happens just preceding failure. Your arms begin to shake, your form deteriorates, and you begin training yourself neurologically to do something that you don't need to learn—how to lift a weight with your arms shaking. It confuses the system, in other words, which is why lifting to failure may make you bigger muscularly, but it also might make you dumber. Muscularly, of course.

Sets

Like reps, sets are another way to make sure you aren't lifting too much weight. The standard advice to lift two to three sets is a way to ensure a volume of work sufficient to develop new strength in as many fibers possible. But it also is a way to make sure you are lifting a light enough weight to protect your joints as well. That said, for most people new to lifting, one set of a resistance exercise is enough to develop new strength. To build upon a foundation of basic strength, however, you need to challenge as many muscle fibers as possible, and to do that, two to three sets are preferable. To obtain your multiple sets, you can either work through your lifts sequentially in multiple cycles through a circuit, or you can stack your sets one after another. All things being equal, the two are the same. An exercise circuit done three times around the horn yields the same strength gains as the same exercises lifted in three-set clusters.

"As long as you're lifting the same load for the same number of times, the net effect on your strength will be similar whether you do them in sets in a row or broken up by other lifts" says William Kraemer, former president of the National Strength and Conditioning Association and co-author of *Designing Resistance Training Programs* (Human Kinetics Press, 2004). "You may get more local muscle endurance if you do them together and keep the rest periods under two minutes. But the disadvantage is you have to be ready for it or you won't be able to get the same load up as many times consecutively."

There are practical and some physiological benefits to both working through a circuit and clustering your sets. Circuit training, or moving from one set of one lift, to one set of another lift, two to three times around the horn, allows you to do more work in less time; for example, you can use recovery time needed from a pushing exercise to do a pulling exercise instead of sitting on the bench waiting for your muscles to get ready to lift the same movement again. By moving quickly from one lift to another, you can also get an aerobic workout. But knocking off clusters of sets on the same exercises—especially working toward shorter recovery times between the sets—trains your muscles for sports that require repeated strength bouts in succession. There are practical reasons to cluster sets

together as well: Who wants to keep reloading the weight stack when you can load it once, do your multiple sets in one block, and be done with it for the day? And who can guarantee that you will be able to jump on the next lift in a circuit with no one else using it? These factors point to an advantage for circuit training when you are in the early stages of a strength-training plan, when you are doing 15–20 repetitions of a lift, and usually only one set. For absolute beginners this could take up much of your first year of training. But the advantage shifts to clustering your sets together once you begin moving into loads that you can lift 10–12 repetitions at a time.

Core Engagement

It seems like you can't open up a magazine anymore without hearing about core strength. From books to videos to the Pilates fitness craze, more and more training has been structured around the idea that fitness emanates from a strong abdominal core. Most people generally think the core is merely the abs, the "six-pack" you can spot with the naked eye, and tend to think that training the core comes down to knocking off a bunch of crunches at the start of the workout. In reality, the abdominal muscles also known as the six-pack are but a superficial layer of muscles on top of the true core, which is a veritable corset of overlapping muscle that stabilizes the pelvic region, links the upper and lower body, and anchors the strength movements of your limbs with a solid pillar of support. Strengthening the core is not so much addressed by crunches, but rather an overall emphasis on ground-based movements that place you on your feet with your back unsupported, such as lunges, squats, standing cable presses, and abdominal rotations. Also, sitting or lying on a stability ball requires your midsection to constantly stabilize your body weight, and this also builds core strength.

To ensure your core is engaged, strengthened, and protecting your spine, many trainers recommend you proceed with most resistance work by consciously pulling your belly button to your spine prior to the initiation of any standing work effort. They argue that this causes you to set the abdominal support muscles that lie beneath your six-pack—the two layers of angular muscle known as the external and internal obliques, and the third layer running sideways known as the transverse abdominals. Others argue that the so-called "drawing-in-maneuver" is an unnatural distraction, and not very sensible at that. If a boxer is about to take a hit to the breadbasket, drawing in his belly might simply expose his organs to worse abuse. All that being said, it seems like becoming mindful of your core and its importance as a strong link for any standing effort is a valuable part of any strength training practice.

Spotters

Spotters—lifting partners or other bystanders enlisted to help oversee your completion of a difficult lift safely—are there less to serve the obvious safety purpose of ensuring a barbell doesn't come crashing down on your throat, than to enable you to challenge yourself with more weight than you might confidently push all alone. In this sense spotters enable you to work until form failure on lifts leave you in a compromising position. Spotters are

helpful with the bench press, military press, and squat, though those not shooting for maximum strength development often can use lighter weights (such as dumbbells) and work fine on their own. Always tell your spotter how many repetitions you are trying to lift in a set. The code of the gym says you need to say yes when someone asks you for a spot, and if they begin to fail, to provide only the lightest assistance, both verbal and physical, required to help them complete the lift. Of course, like the exit row seat on the airplane, you are free to decline the request if you feel you may be unable to carry out the duties.

Breathing

It's hard to believe you need instructions on how to breathe, but strength training has a way of making a lot of natural occurrences seem alien. Inhale before a lift, and exhale as you do the work of moving the resistance, also known as the sticking point. All that's happening here is you are making sure your muscles are fully engaged at the point when you need them most, and this happens to coincide with having a full breath. If this all seems too complex to be natural, keep in mind that correct breathing is likely something you will adopt intuitively.

Duration and Frequency

The honest ones all will tell you they aren't crazy about lifting weights. It can be tedious, the music is often bad, the gear looks like it has other people's colds, it's almost always nicer outside, and the company smells. But they do it and they get on with it, make it worthwhile, and get out.

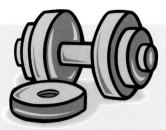

MUSCLE SORENESS

For most of us, post-workout strength-training recovery requires 36 hours of downtime, which is why most strength regimens send you to the weight room every other day. Chances are that in the beginning of a training plan you might need more than a day off to stop feeling sore, especially if you are over 30 or have managed to put yourself through any so-called eccentric overload contractions, muscle-lengthening strength exercises like slow letting down of more weight than you can push, and which can create extended periods of soreness known as delayed onset muscle soreness, or DOMS (see below). For those needing a five-day-a-week fix, there are ways to lift Monday through Friday. You can alternate your work assignments so that one set of muscles are built on one day while another is built the following day, though they become less easy to differentiate the more you veer from training your anatomy and turn toward training movements. Because you are never doing the kind of isolation capable of causing overload, you can generally work your core seven days a week.

Soreness is generally divided into two categories, garden-variety soreness signaling the aftereffects of exertion, and that more vexing sort believed to be due to microtears and inflammation deep in the muscle. We have all have had the nice sore feeling you get after a good workout, but DOMS feels worse, and can last for weeks. DOMS is exceedingly well correlated with so-called eccentric contractions, or the type of work you do in letting a weight down slowly.

DOMS makes you weaker while the muscle is healing, so working out through it won't make you any stronger, and may delay healing. Working with lighter weights has been shown to be of little help in shortening DOMS either. A study from Greece that was published in the *Journal of Strength and Conditioning Research* did show a benefit in reducing pain from DOMS through taking 400mg of ibuprofen every 8 hours, though doing so didn't help the subjects return to normal strength any sooner. The good news is you will be less likely to get so sore the next time you try an eccentric workout.

Some even use the drabness of the gym as motivation. Joe Decker, holder of the Guinness Book of World Records 24-Hour Physical Fitness Challenge title for a day spent doing 1,100 push-ups, 3,000 crunches, and lifting over a quarter of a million pounds, puts it like this: "I'd rather be on the trail. Forty-five minutes to an hour in the weight room and I need to get out of there or I'm starting to lose my focus." And he's supposedly the world's fittest man.

How does he keep himself on task? "If I do an easy set of ten, I stop and tell myself 'why come in here and waste your time?' Then I go back and do them right."

In other words, there are plenty of great reasons why you want to stay busy around weights, working with purpose and focus on the goal at hand. For most of us, that means trying to get out of the weight room in an hour. When you factor in the down time spent waiting for muscles to recover, gear to become available, and the extra sets needed to build new muscle, that can sometimes turn into an hour and a half. But it's a grim place. You're going to want to do whatever you can to keep it under an hour. Because of your need for recovery, there is little value to strength training for more than two to three days a week, and if you are new to it, two days a week can be more than enough time spent getting sore in the gym.

Recovery

Workout charts stagger weight training and recovery days with nuanced complexity, but all you really need to know is that you can't go back to lift again until your muscles start feeling better. Provided you have worked against enough resistance to experience overload, your muscles take on a gentle ache after lifting, caused by the buildup of lactic acid and minuscule tears in the muscle cells that signal the fact that your muscles are getting stronger. You may push the plates in the gym, but strength is created while home on the couch. Your recovering muscles always need a day off.

Working out with a sore muscle won't necessarily hurt you—except for those gym rats who return to the scene of the crime without a day off so repeatedly they invite the burnout known as overtraining—but it probably won't help you get any stronger either. Working out with sore muscles delays muscular rebuilding, and even if it didn't, your muscles simply couldn't push enough resistance while sore to make many gains anyway. You can work through moderate soreness—which should feel nothing like pain, however—and sometimes the working out will bring enough blood to the area to make the soreness go away. But for heavier soreness, it usually means you need a little more time for recovery, in which case you have to wait out the soreness. Listen to your body, not your training chart.

A MOVEMENT-BASED STRENGTH PLAN

The weight room only seeks to stage with weights or your body weight the small number of things that you can accomplish with the human form. All we have are two arms, two legs, and a waist that extends and rotates. You can organize your workouts around, say, your chest and legs, but basically it is the utter simplicity of how we move that best explains weight lifting in a meaningful way.

Your body can push, pull, rotate, bend, step, and squat. The easiest way to make sure your training plan is both functional and complete is to organize your lifts according to these movements, rather than your Latin-named body parts, and to balance your movements, with work that targets its oppositional movement. For instance, after you push with your upper body, turn to pulling with your upper body. After you push a weight over your head, pull a weight downward from over your head. Move from lifts targeting the largest muscles to those targeting smaller muscles. Rest sufficiently between training sessions to let your body adapt to the stress.

Once you begin to think about your lifts along the lines of their basic movements—working as much as possible with body weight, pairing them with an oppositional movement, and eventually adding a destabilized version to make the lift even more functional, and for those willing, proceeding to a maximum-strength version with dumbbells or barbells—structuring your weight-lifting time becomes far more instinctive, sport-specific, and improvisational, lending variety, functionality, and creativity to your workouts. The following section highlights a representative sample of two to three strength-training options for all the basic movements, but the menu of choices is limitless.

Nine Basic Strength Movements

Human biomechanics limit most of our work to variations on a few basic movements: pushing and pulling with the arms, chest, shoulders, and back; stepping or squatting with your hips, rear, and legs; bending-extending at your waist and lower

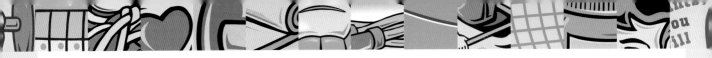

YOU CAN THINK OF THE **PUSHING** MOVEMENTS LIKE THIS:

Pushing movement type	Basic pushing exercises	Complex pushing exercises
Forward Pushing	Push-ups, bench press, seated chest press, medicine ball throw, wall push-up	Push-ups and throw on ball, bench press with dumbbells and on ball, chest press standing with cable
Upward Pushing	Seated dumbbell press, standing dumbbell press	Seated on ball and with dumbbells, standing press with dumbbells and on one leg
Downward Pushing	Dips, dumbbell tricep kickback, cable tricep extensions.	Overhead tricep extension from a prone position on ball

YOU CAN THINK OF THE **PULLING** MOVEMENTS LIKE THIS:

Pulling movement type	Basic pulling exercises	Complex pulling exercises
Forward Pulling	Seated row, dumbbell row	Standing cable row, dumbbell row on ball
Upward Pulling	Upright rows, barbell curls, shrug	Seated on ball, dumbbell curl
Downward Pulling	Lat pull-down, chin-up, wide-grip pull-up, V-handle pull-up	Lat pull-down from ball, alternating dual cable lat pull-down

YOU CAN THINK OF THE **ROTATING** MOVEMENTS LIKE THIS:

Rotating movement type	Basic rotational exercises	Complex rotational exercises
Sideways Rotation	Medicine ball rotation, fitness bar rotation hanging hip rotation, sideway cable rotation	Sideway ball throw, Russian twist on stability ball, lying hip rotation with stability ball
Upward Rotation	Reverse wood chop, dumbbell reach from opposite side	Dumbbell reach with one leg on ball
Downward Rotation	Oblique curl, medicine ball wood chop, cable wood chop, dumbbell chop	Oblique curl on ball

YOU CAN THINK OF THE BENDING MOVEMENTS LIKE THIS:

Bending movement type	Basic bending exercises	Complex bending exercises
Bending	Crunch, overhead medicine ball throw from sit-up	Crunch throw from ball
Extending	Romanian deadlift, Superman, kneeling forward bend and extension	Extension on ball

YOU CAN THINK OF THE STEPPING MOVEMENTS LIKE THIS:

Stepping movement type	Basic stepping exercises	Complex stepping exercises
Forward Stepping	Side lunge, lunge, dumbbell lunge	Forward step down from box, step up to box

AND LAST BUT NOT LEAST, YOU CAN THINK OF THE SQUATTING MOVEMENTS LIKE THIS:

Movement	Basic squatting exercises	Complex squatting exercises
Squatting	Bodyweight squat, barbell squat, dumbbell squat	One-legged bodyweight squat, split-stance barbell squat, leg on ball squat

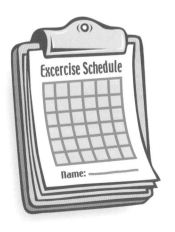

Excercise Schedule

Name:

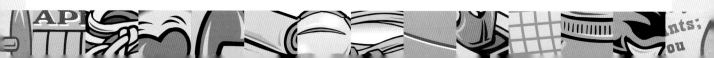

back, and rotating your pelvis. Nearly everything you do in a resistance plan can be organized around these basic movements, and every basic movement can be strengthened in a variety of ways depending upon where you are in your strength development and what your goals are. At best, you probably have enough time in a typical full-body strength workout to train each movement once. If you try to hit them all, you will be more likely to get a balanced workout.

For each of the following nine basic movements that follow you will find a menu of Beginner, Intermediate, and Advanced strength-training options. As a rule, those with little previous strength training will do better by progressing from machine-assisted or modified body-weight options first. Those with better development can consider choosing from body-weight options of lifts and destabilized options. Those with an advanced strength-

training background can benefit from maximum strength options with dumbbells and, if desired (though it is not necessary) barbells. Keep in mind that pushing a lot of weight or building large muscles for their own sake doesn't really have a lot in common with the sort of integrated strength that is called for in many outdoors sports. If you aren't hoping to play in the NFL, there is little reason to train like you are, and plenty of reasons not to, beginning with the declining risk-reward relationship for your joints the more weight you try to push. You can get in fantastic shape simply using your body weight or dumbbells. Proceed with each lift only after a vigorous warm-up that leaves you sweating, and in the case of weighted lifts, with an unweighted set taken through its full range of motion. Rest for 60–90 seconds between each exercise or as long as it takes to get yourself ready for another set.

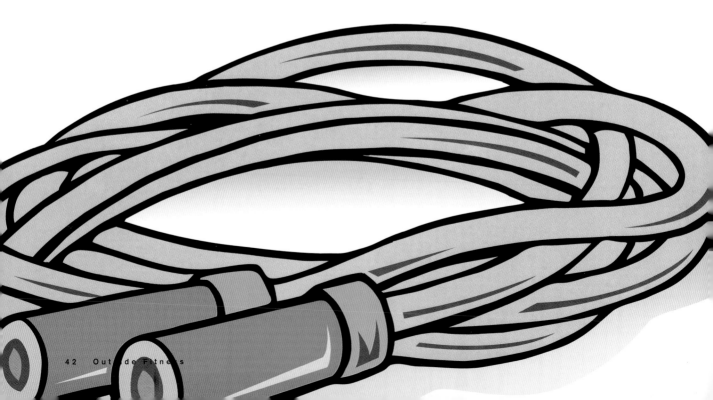

Strength Movement 1: SQUATTING

Squatting is an activity that transfers to sports in the field, from climbing to skiing to skating, and it uses more muscles than most lifts. Because it uses so many muscles, it is good to do your squats early in a workout, while the muscles haven't yet been taxed individually. Few people can even squat their own body weight, much less dumbbells or barbells. For this reason, prior to beginning squat training loaded with dumbbells or barbells you should first be able to simply do multiple, controlled body-weight squats with your fingers laced behind your head ("prisoner squats"). Once your body-weight squatting skills are old hat—maybe you can do 20 in a half minute—progress to squatting with a leg press, dumbbells either at your shoulders or hanging at your sides, and if you still desire more progression, finally to barbells. Loaded squatting puts a lot of force on your spine and knees, two joints that do not come with warranties, so err on the side of underloading and moving slowly in adding more weight. Those with knee or back problems should consider avoiding loaded squats entirely.

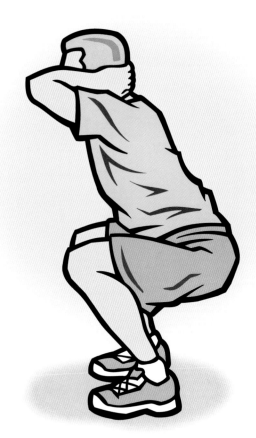

Beginner: Leg Press

Directions: Adjust the sled so your knees are bent at 90-degree angles at rest, keep your rear down, your head back, hold the handles, and push your legs outward in a controlled movement. At the end of your push, take care not to lock your knees.

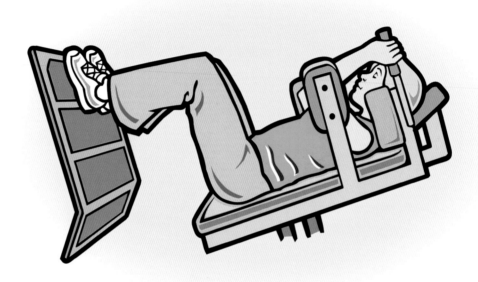

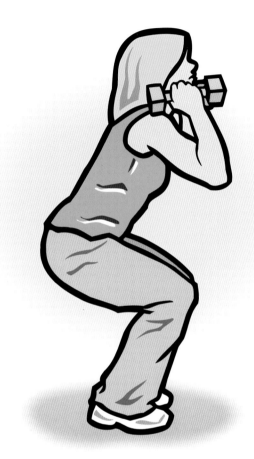

Intermediate: Dumbbell Squat

Directions: With feet shoulder-width apart and your back in a neutral position, hold dumbbells at your sides or up against your shoulders. Squat until your thighs are parallel to the floor, pause, and return to your starting position in a controlled movement.

Advanced: Barbell Squat

Directions: Hold the barbell on your upper back, arms shoulder-width apart and your back in a neutral position. Squat until your thighs are parallel to the floor, pause, and return to your starting position in a controlled movement. Take care not to lock your knees and to keep your head looking forward.

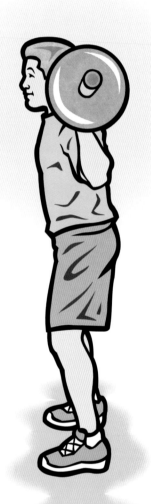

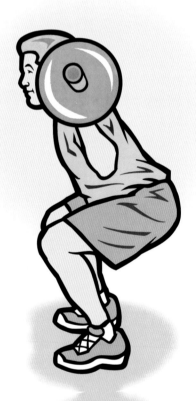

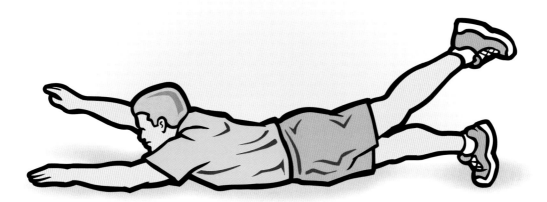

Prone Back Extension ("Superman")

Strength Movement 2: BENDING AND EXTENDING

Extending is vital to everything from launching a mountain bike to lifting a pack from your campsite. The Sun Salutation series in the flexibility chapter can help build your body-weight bending and extending strength, but to develop greater extension strength, try a stability ball extension, prone back extension, or a Romanian dead lift using dumbbells. For those susceptible to low back injury—and there's little way of knowing you are susceptible until the day you bend over to pick up a newspaper and feel your body start sending Eddie Van Halen guitar solos through your sciatic nerve pathways—holding a weight and bending with a bent or straight back are both more risky than any benefit from the movement justifies. It's good to have strong lower back extension strength (the ability to pull yourself, and possibly a weight, upright) but you really only need it in conjunction with the bending of your ankles, knees, and hips. Chances are, with bent knees and strong quads, you can pull most objects from the floor without ever having to bend your back more than a modestly forward-leaning angle.

Beginner: Prone Back Extension ("Superman")

Directions: Laying face down on a mat, lift one arm and the opposite leg upward, hold for three seconds, and return back down in a controlled movement. Repeat on other side. You can also do this exercise by lifting both arms and legs simultaneously. Do not extend farther than feels comfortable.

Intermediate: Stability-Ball Back Extension

Directions: Stabilizing your weight with your feet hooked under a stable bench or with legs spread and weight on toes, place your stomach and hips on the stability ball, cross your arms at the chest, and bend at the waist with a straight back as far as the ball lets you. Return to your starting position, careful to stop your extension when your body becomes straight.

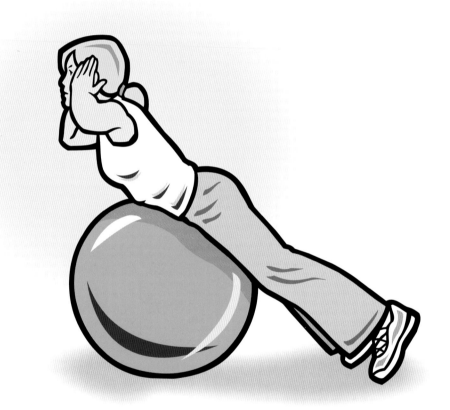

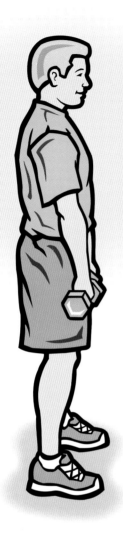
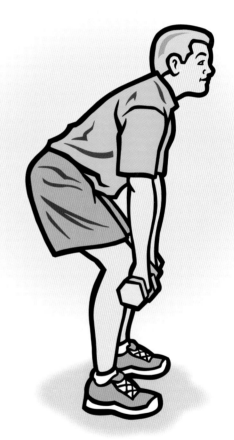

Advanced: Bent-Knee Dead Lift with Dumbbells

Directions: Holding two dumbbells at mid-thigh level, with your back straight and your head up, drop carefully through your heels, knees, and hips to shin height, then lift the weights up into a standing position, arms hanging at your thighs. You can also bend your knees enough to lower the weights to the floor, but much of that work duplicates the squat. Keep your lower back straight.

Strength Movement 3: FORWARD STEPPING

Stepping movements are modifications of squatting movements, and are highly functional for out-door sports. You need controlled knee, glute, and hip stabilization with your leg in extended positions for sports ranging from cross-country skiing to trekking to telemarking. To reduce knee strain, you want to avoid letting your knee cross the plane of the front of your foot when forward stepping. As with other strength movements, start out simply stepping with your own body weight before moving up to dumbbells. To make body-weight lunges even more knee-sparing, simply repeat a set of body-weight squats with your legs stationed in a stepping position, then repeat from the other side. Barbells are an advanced option for those who have built up the stabilization strength from body-weight work and who want to build increased strength, but are not necessary.

Beginner: Body-Weight Lunge

Start with legs split front and back, and squat so the front thigh is parallel to the floor then return to standing. After set is complete, repeat with other leg forward.

Intermediate: Dumbbell Lunge

Directions: Holding dumbbells at your sides, step forward with one leg into a lunge so that your front thigh is parallel to the floor and forward knee is behind the plane of your forward foot. Stabilize your back leg with your weight on the forefoot and point your back knee to the floor. To make this a complex movement, curl the dumbbells to your shoulders. Step back and repeat. When reps are finished, repeat with the other leg, or alternate legs.

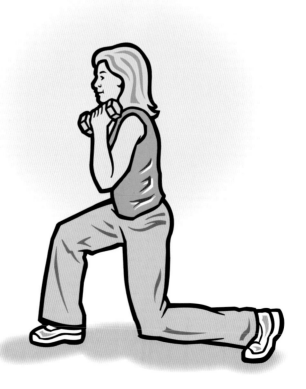

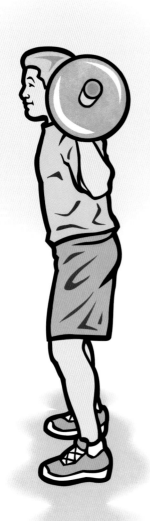
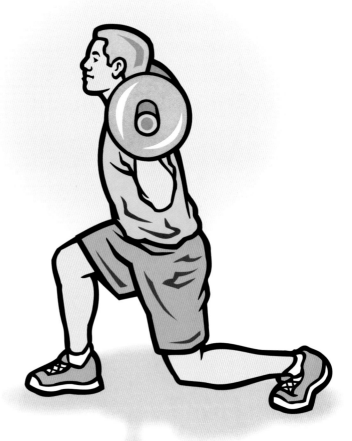

Advanced: Barbell Lunge

Holding a barbell at the top of your back, step forward with one leg into a lunge. Step back and repeat. When reps are finished, repeat with the other leg.

Strength Movement 4: ROTATING

You rotate with every throw and paddle stroke you take, as well as any time you twist to change directions or make a turn down a mogul field. Various sports and forms of manual labor all call for rotational movements, yet these are strengthened only rarely. Increasingly, trainers are recognizing the need to train the transverse abdominals in a functional manner. The primary objectives for reducing back strain in twisting movements are to: load weight conservatively, lead with the pelvis, minimize bending, and leave your back heel free to turn with your hips. Those with back problems should stick to side-to-side rotations. Whenever rotating, shoot for control, not poundage.

Beginner: Oblique Crunch

Directions: Lie on your back, with your fingertips at the side of your head, lift your shoulders from the floor, and rotate to alternate sides at the top of each movement.

Intermediate: Medicine-Ball Rotation or Lateral Cable Pull

Directions: Standing with a medicine ball in your hands, lead with your pelvis and rotate your abdomen from side to side in controlled movements and let your shoulders follow. Leave your following heel free to turn with the rotation. To train this movement with cables, stand with a cable machine at mid-side, turn with heels free to grab the cable with your opposite arm, and turn your pelvis to bring it 180 degrees across your body. Return to the starting point in a controlled movement and repeat.

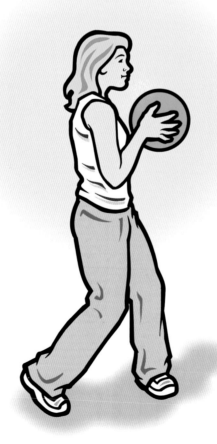

Advanced: Cable Wood Chop or Reverse Wood Chop

Directions: For the wood chop, which is more of a sport-affiliated movement, hold a cable with light weight outside one shoulder at arm's length. Rotate your pelvis, keep your arms in a triangle and pull the weight with your core, finishing with a slight bend to move toward the outside of the other side of your waist. Let your heels rotate with the movement and repeat the set from the other side when you are finished. For the reverse wood chop, which is a more work-affiliated movement, start facing the weight and bring it from the outside of one leg to the outside of the reverse side shoulder.

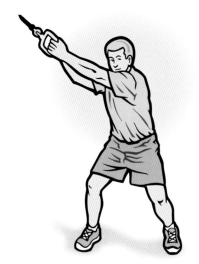
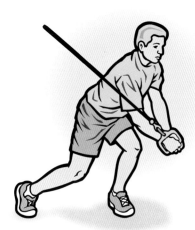

Cable Wood Chop

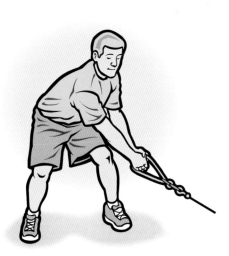
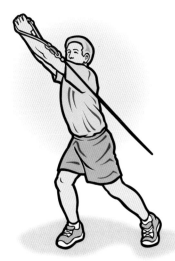

Reverse Wood Chop

Strength Movement 5: FORWARD PULLING

Pulling movements originate in the upper back, front of the arms, and shoulders and are invaluable for rowing, climbing, cycling, and other outdoor sports. You can pull things toward you (open-chain movements useful for activities like rowing) or you can pull your body toward something immobile (closed-chain movements found in climbing and gymnastics). Developing pulls is also a corrective to staying balanced in your musculature given all the pushing strength development that goes on in weight rooms. You can pull from forward, below, and overhead. Despite the bodybuilding popularity of upward pulls like the bicep curl and upright row, the most functional pulling movements are those from forward and overhead. Because they provide the anchor for pulls from forward, the muscles of your core are activated in forward pulls, whether they are based on a knee, ball, or bench, making these not only specific to the rowing sports but functional for lifting tasks where your body is extended over its base of support.

Beginner: Incline Pull-Up

Directions: Lower a bar on a rack to a point that enables you to pull yourself upward. The higher you place the bar, the lighter the load on your pulling muscles. Your feet should be positioned in front of your body, and your body should form a straight line at an angle from the bar. Pull yourself to the bar, and descend back to a starting point with your arms straight but without elbows locked.

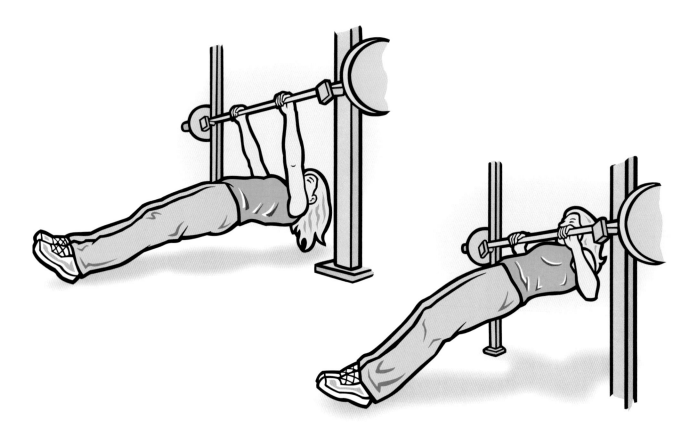

Intermediate: Stability-Ball Dumbbell Row

Directions: Resting one straight arm on a stability ball, with your leg stepping forward on the same side knee, row a dumbbell from a hanging position to your side. Return to a hanging position and repeat, before switching to do the exercise from the other side.

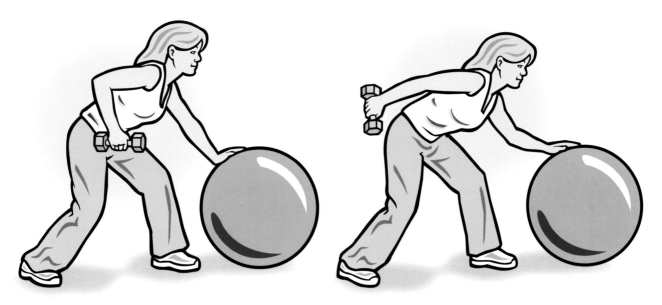

Advanced: Dumbbell Row

Directions: The basic row operates by supporting one arm and knee on a bench, then hanging the weight from the other arm and rowing it upward. But how often do you lift something while kneeling on a bench? You can make it more functional by simply extending your knee into a lunge and resting your non-rowing arm on your knee. Pull the weight to your side for the target number of reps, and repeat on the other side.

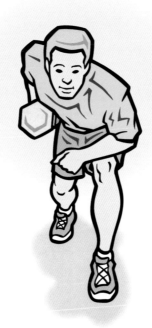

Strength Movement 6: OVERHEAD PULLING

You may not have much occasion, outside of the task of building your lats, to pull something down-ward toward you (it requires pulleys and cables). But being able to pull yourself upward (the closed-chain form of overhead pulling) is needed not just for cresting a climbing wall, but for a balanced level of control over your body, whether climbing a ladder, tree, or rope.

Beginner: Lat Pull-Down

Directions: Grab the bar at shoulder-width, lean back slightly, pull your shoulder blades together, and contract the muscles of the upper back to pull the bar to your chest. When you are finished, release upward in a controlled movement.

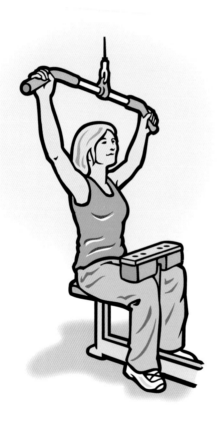

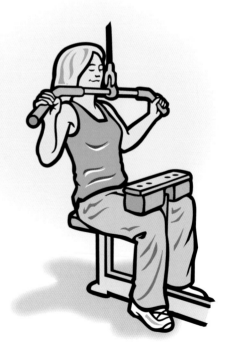

Intermediate: Chin-Up or Incline Chin-Up

Directions: Grab the bar with your palms facing you, arms in front of your shoulders, and pull your body up until your chin passes the bar. Descend to as much of a full hang as possible without letting your elbows lock. If this is too challenging, practice with an incline chin-up—like an incline pull-up but with your palms facing you.

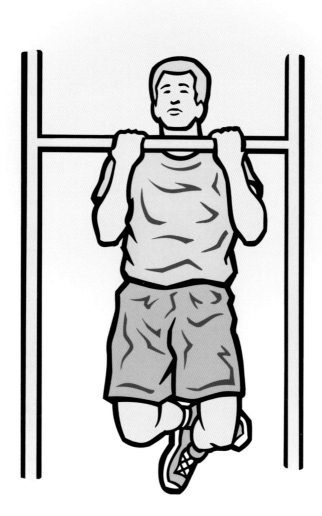

Advanced: Pull-Up

Directions: Grab the bar with palms facing forward and arms wider than shoulder-width. Pull your shoulder blades together, pull yourself up until your chest touches the bar, and lower yourself to a starting position as close to a full hang as possible without locking elbows. For an even greater challenge, move arms farther apart on the bar.

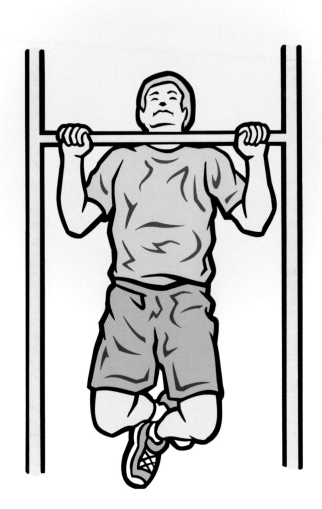

Strength Movement 7: FORWARD PUSHING

Pushing extends your limbs away from your body. Since it builds the muscles you see in the mirror, upper-body pushing is highly valued in the weight room, but it is only marginally important to outdoor activities. (You actually pull a lot more often—especially during paddling, mountain biking, cycling, windsurfing, and climbing.) When it comes to forward pushes, thanks to gravity you can push your body away from a fixed surface (as in a push-up) and you can push an object away from your body (as in a dumbbell press), but both are merely preparatory to pushing something forward while standing (as in a standing cable press). Once you progress beyond machine presses or push-up-based body-weight work—which is no small accomplishment—dumbbells are the best way to start developing forward pushing strength, because they force you to develop symmetrical strength (a barbell can hide a side dominance), and make the lift challenge the stabilizing muscles of your shoulder.

Beginner: Seated Machine Press or Push-Up

Directions: For the machine press, sit and push the handles outward, and take care not to lock your elbows.

For the push-up, start in a position with your arms spread shoulder-width apart, your weight on your hands and toes, core engaged, and elbows straight but not locked. Keep your back in neutral, descend in controlled movements until your elbows reach 90 degrees, and return to the starting position without locking your elbows. If push-ups are too challenging, try them from your knees, or while leaning against a wall, against the back of a stable chair, or against an elevated step on a staircase. To make this more challenging, elevate your feet or place them on a stability ball.

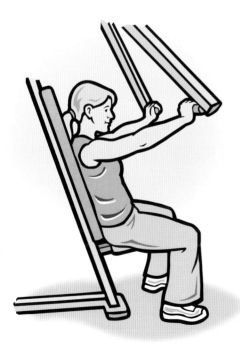

Seated Machine Press

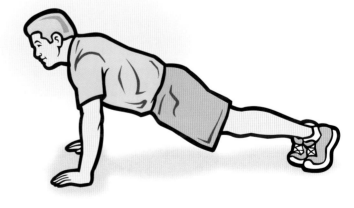

Push-Up

Intermediate: Stability-Ball Chest Press

Directions: With dumbbells in hands, roll from seated to a position with your shoulders on the ball, your hips raised, and core engaged. Lower the dumbbells toward your shoulders with your elbows pointing outward, then press them upward, keeping your arms over your shoulders, and repeat in smooth, controlled movements.

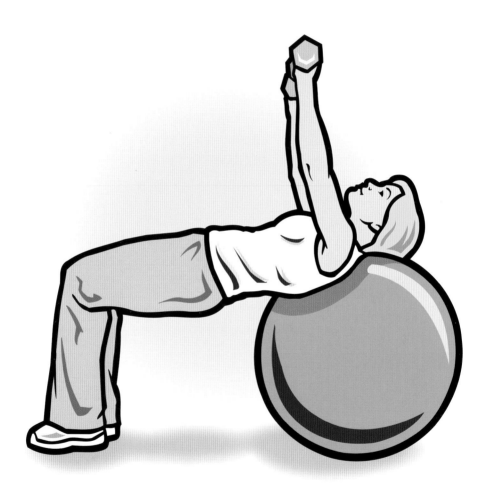

Advanced: Dumbbell or Barbell Bench Press

Directions: Lower the weights at a controlled pace to a position just above your chest (for those concerned about shoulder stress, stop at a point with elbows at 90 degrees). Pause, and then push upward. Do not lock elbows. It is best to bench press dumbbells though barbells can eventually become necessary for those seeking maximum strength development.

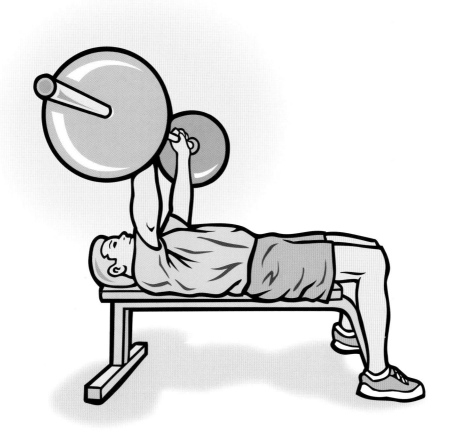

Strength Movement 8: OVERHEAD PUSHING

Overhead pushing is an activity the body-building press may file under "shoulders," but it is called upon anytime you load a bike or canoe atop a car. To accentuate shoulder development, the weight room offers backrests for those doing overhead pushes, but outdoors you simply need to push above you only that level of weight you can elevate while standing. Because these exercises can put strain on your shoulders, they should be done with dumbbells, to keep your movements free and your weight in control. Those with shoulder problems should stick to pushing in movements that do not raise their arms overhead.

Beginner: Seated Overhead Machine Press

Directions: Push the handles upward until your arms are extended but your elbows are not locked. Lower the weight carefully and repeat.

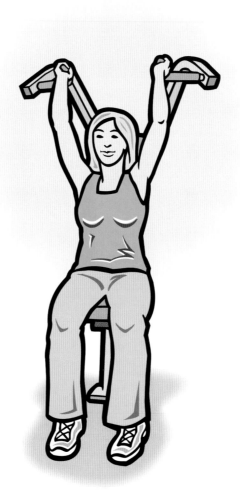

Intermediate: Stability-Ball Dumbbell Press

Directions: Seated on the stability ball, with your back in neutral and thighs parallel to floor, hold dumbbells at shoulder height, palms facing the sides of your face. Push upward, allowing your wrists to turn 90 degrees, to a point where your palms face outward.

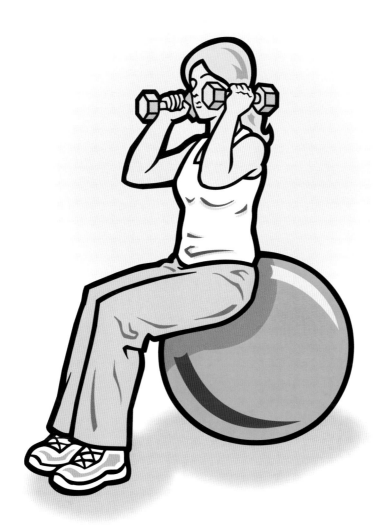

Advanced: Dumbbell Press

Directions: Begin with dumbbells at shoulder height, palms facing inward. Push upward, allowing palms to turn outward at the top of extension.

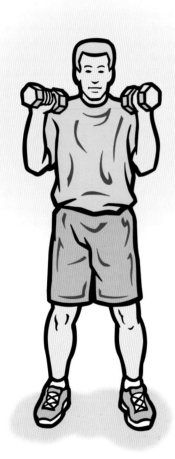

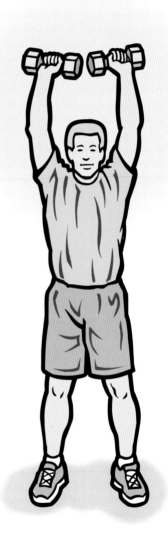

Strength Movement 9: DOWNWARD PUSHING

Downward pushing strength is the force required to clear the lip of a ledge, to finish a kayak stroke, and to swing your body over a fallen tree. It is the opposite of a bicep curl, both in its biomechanics and genuine usefulness.

Beginner: Tricep Kickback

Directions: Propping an arm and knee on a bench, your other arm holding a dumbbell to your side with a bent elbow, extend your arm to push the dumbbell behind you. When reps are finished, repeat with the other arm.

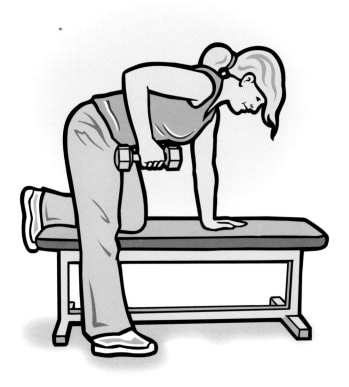

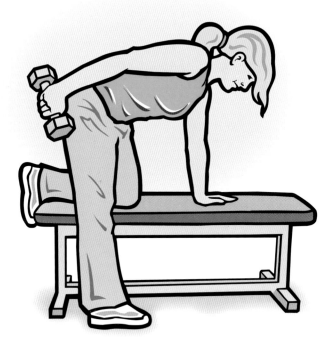

Intermediate: Stability-Ball Tricep Extension

Directions: This is the same as tricep kickback, but you support your weight on a stability ball.

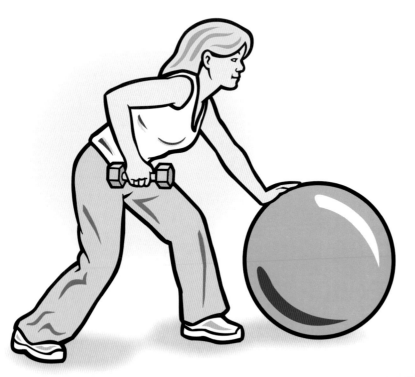

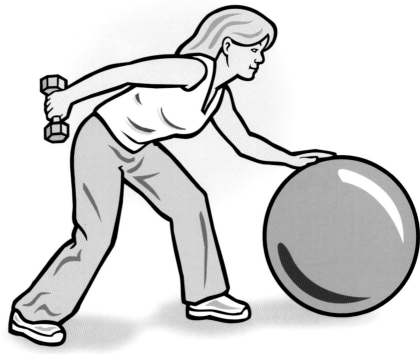

Advanced: Tricep Extension

Directions: Standing at a cable machine with your elbows at your sides, grab the handle at chest height and straighten your arms downward to push the weight to your waist. Release the weight upward with control and repeat. This can also be done by lowering your body weight against a chair seat, with arms positioned behind your back. Both should be avoided by those with shoulder injuries.

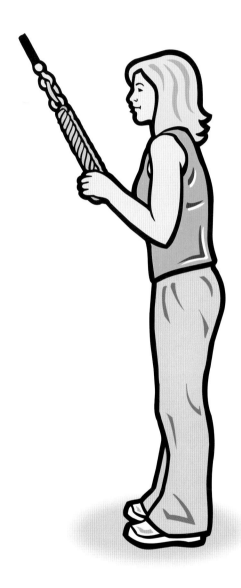

STRENGTH IS INDIVIDUAL

Chances are, different readers want different things from strength and very little about what you do to develop strength will stay the same throughout your lifetime. Those who are highly fit and have the energy to sleep off the soreness might like building mass and raw strength, then buying the new clothing required to encase their bigger muscles. Those unmoved by this goal might take more interest in using dumbbells and stability balls to locate new biomechanical struggles to untangle and master. Still others might be amazed at the potential and functionality of developing strength simply through pitting their limbs against their own body weight. All are called strength training, and all are different. But if you take away one idea from the strength-training ideas and exercises offered in this chapter, let it be to approach strength as a way to do specific work, rather than building specific muscles. Do so and give yourself a platform to redesign and reformat exercises of your choosing throughout the coming years, as your work and goals change with you.

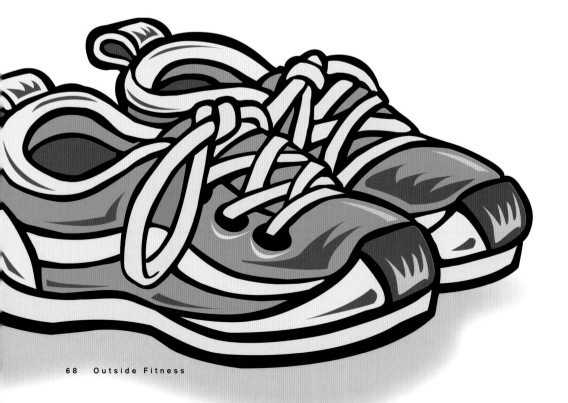

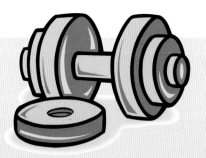

WHAT'S THE DEAL WITH WEIGHT-LIFTING BELTS?

If you're confused about the utility of those wide leather straps by the squat rack, you're not alone. Thanks to a recent Mayo Clinic study published in the *Journal of Strength and Conditioning Research,* we now know that the majority of people interviewed in at least one health club were wearing weight belts at the wrong time, for the wrong reasons. The National Strength and Conditioning Association recommends wearing them only for near-maximal or maximal weights (if at all) and then only for lifts that expose the lower spine to compression. The reason for all the above "onlys" is that the more you buttress your core externally, the more you weaken it internally. Ideally, you want to develop your core into its own weight belt.

The study found that 90 percent of current belt users thought wearing the belt would help prevent injury, and 22 percent thought doing so helped improve performance, when in fact the research literature is divided on both questions. The study also found that over half of all belt users used them on lighter loads, which is counterindicated. Moreover, some users said they would use the belt during exercises like the bench press, where, done correctly, the lower back is just fine on its own, thank you very much. One guy even used it during his cardio, perhaps just for his very own little treadmill/back-weakening session. None of this should be surprising, given the way employees wear them around the store at big hardware outlets. But the casual use of a tool designed for guys like "Pocket Hercules," the diminutive Turkish Olympic weightlifter, does indicate, as the authors suggested, an area for better education.

chapter 4
FLEXIBILITY

FLEXIBILITY IS THE RANGE OF MOTION your muscles and tendons allow your joints. Unless you've experienced the debilitating wrath of some **LATIN-NAMED MUSCLE** in the small of your back dancing into spasm, or unless you have accumulated

enough 10-mile runs to lie awake at night from hamstrings as tight as piano strings, chances are you'll never feel your muscles and tendons tightening. You will just notice that you have begun moving funny: that for five years now you have been squatting instead of bending; that you have stopped looking over your shoulder when you change lanes; that something is seriously wrong with the yoga instructor telling you to clasp your hands behind your back, lean forward, and pull them into an arrow pointing at the knees of the person in front of you. Are you supposed to be able to do that?

There are a host of movements for which you are designed—and that you need to call on if you are to be effective in outdoor mayhem—that the routines of a modern life never seem to require. These include: folding your frame at the waist to set your nose between your knees (needed to untangle a snagged fly, not needed when driving, watching television, eating, or

sleeping); lacing your fingers, counter-rotating your wrists, extending your elbows, and turning your palms toward the ceiling (needed while portaging a canoe; not needed when exchanging a DVD at Best Buy); and simply sitting cross-legged with your other foot under your thigh for once.

Thanks to our endless repetition of the same few everyday movements, over time our bodies distort to enable the shortest path between the same three or four activities.

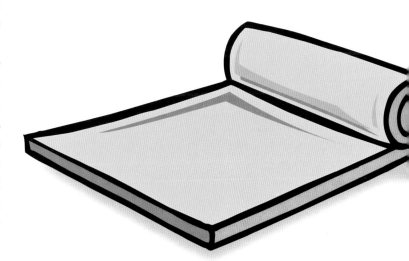

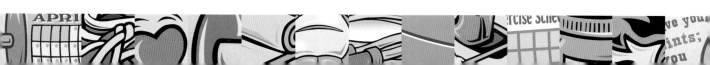

That's the theory: In practice our shoulders, pelvis, neck, hips, and ankles all begin to lose their range of motion, all of which invites injury and reduces our performance out on the trail, stream, or wall. How exactly does this happen?

YOU STARTED OUT IN LIFE AS LIMBER AS A SWAMI

Stretching may seem like an alternative lifestyle choice, a calming respite for the leisure class, but consider the problems it addresses, and you quickly conclude that stretching is much more than a luxury. Stretching is a necessary corrective needed to restore what nature intended.

We didn't used to be so tight. Our muscles and joints started out life with their widest possible range of motion. Just observe the untrained flexibility of an infant laying on the changing table—quads casually raised to chest by his own power when most of us would be lucky to pull them to vertical—to appreciate the extent to which the range of motion of the human skeleton can become realigned through decades of selective muscle shortening. We get tighter as we age, but far from being an inevitable part of life, our progressively shrinking range of motion is highly reversible with a regular flexibility program.

Flexibility is not only natural but democratic. You don't have to pay for a hot yoga class to bend like a swami—just from ripping off shingles, many roofers can fold like ballerinas. Fortunately, the wide range of motion required for the strength exercises listed in the previous chapter will do its part in establishing new expectations for how far your body can bend, extend, and rotate. By holding your body weight in extended positions, the active stretches and yoga sequences described in this chapter will make your body strong in ways not possible through traditional strength training. Together that will make for less of the tightness that accompanies modern life, fewer of the compensatory movements we undertake accommodate tight muscles (and the injuries these compensatory movements can bring about), and more of the range of motion needed to enable you to perform better in the field.

EVERY TIGHT MUSCLE PULLS A DIFFERENT MUSCLE LOOSE

Muscle tightening wouldn't be such a big deal if the problem was confined to just one or two affected muscles, but muscles are a complex rigging of opposed pairs, and this linked system passes changes in one muscle on to others. Nearly every muscle is either a flexor (puller) or an extensor (pusher) holding each other in place, and in shortening a muscle you invariably cause a loosening of its partner on the other side of your body. Your chest, for example, becomes tight only in concert with the loosening of your upper back. Your hamstrings become tight only in concert with the loosening of butt and lower back. Your calves become tight by the loosening of your shins. Stretching helps reduce the muscular asymmetry of one-dimensional training.

"People think that training gets you in shape. Training gets you out of shape," says Beryl Bender Birch, internationally renowned American yoga teacher and lecturer and author of a pair of books on Ashtanga yoga, and the person credited with inventing the now vernacular term "power yoga." "You can see it immediately. Because their range of motion is so shut down, a lot of weight lifters can't access the strength they've spent so much time developing," she says. "Others are in perfect shape for their sport, and a nanosecond away from exploding somewhere. And the better they are at their sport, the more time it takes to undo it."

Birch is a believer that you have to be soft to be hard—flexible to be strong. It is a mantra she settled on several years ago after teaching a class to the U. S. Nordic Ski Team and finding out the best athletes in the world were so tight in the ankles, back, and quads that they had to phone in sick the day after their first stretch class. "Most athletes worry if they start undoing the tightness they will lose performance," says Birch. "In fact it's the opposite. Becoming more flexible enables you to push the envelope further, to amp up the training."

THE BASICS OF FLEXIBILITY TRAINING

While it has long been characterized as something you do as part of getting ready to work out, flexibility training offers much more when given its own block of time in a training plan. You can train flexibility every day of the week, or just one day a week, but take the time to learn about its method and you stand a much better chance of giving it a permanent place in your training repertoire.

Get Warm

We know we stretch more readily when warm, but we also know this is true not for the reasons we once thought. Our muscles are both elastic and plastic. They can be extended longer than their regular length (elasticity), and if you do that enough they will stay longer (plasticity). We used to think that like taffy, our muscles cells themselves became more viscous (or fluid) when warm, until someone did the math and realized we never get our muscles warm enough to make them physically more stretchy. It turns out the reason we can stretch more easily when warmed up is that warm muscles are more tolerant neurologically to the discomfort of being stretched. They handle the pain better.

It turns out there is something about pain—physically, not mentally—that makes it the limiting factor to getting a good stretch. None of this should be taken to mean you should push a stretch to the point of pain, because nothing could be further from the truth. It means that warming up is a safe way to mask pain enough that your muscles will agree neurologically to stretch. Warming up also increases the energy the muscle can absorb prior to failing while being stretched. To increase the range of motion at which your muscles tighten due to stretching, spend 5–10 minutes briskly walking, cycling, or rowing.

Forget All That Business about Stretching Before a Workout

Now that you know why to stretch, and the importance of getting warm to getting a good stretch, this would traditionally be the place where you read about the Importance of Stretching before Every Workout, to Help Prevent Injuries. Except for one thing: It appears this cornerstone of training dogma is incorrect. Stretching is vital to reducing injuries in general. It resets the structural imbalances that lead to injury and helps build the range of motion necessary to avoid falls. That said, it appears that stretching before a workout not only fails to reduce your chances of getting injured in the ensuing workout, it may even increase them.

Researchers recently compared groups who stretched prior to a workout to those who did not. The stretching groups fared no better in the ensuing workout, injury-wise, than those who did not stretch, and in some cases they fared worse. Sports injuries tend to result from the same factors: poor take-offs and landings, and sudden plants and turns on structurally unsupported joints. In other words, injuries arise from planting, landing, and slowing, none of which are affected by the short-term benefits of a stretching session. Researchers can't even state for certain that stretchy muscles are less likely to rupture, a fear underlying much of the advice to stretch before you train—some believe it is the amount of force you absorb, as opposed to the maximum attainable length of your muscle, that determines when it quits stretching and begins to tear.

All the preceding points address the unlikelihood that pre-workout stretching really prevents injuries in an ensuing workout. As for the possibility that pre-workout stretching could actually do the reverse and lead to more injuries in the ensuing hour in the weight room, start with this: Stretching is work. It makes your muscles both more tired and less responsive. In so doing, stretching is no different than a pre-workout trail run; it can create the immediate muscular condition where your glycogen-drained limbs will be less likely to step up when you need them, and thus give rise to exhaustion-based injury. Aside from just making you tired, pre-workout stretching could cause you to use the wrong muscles in a lift or movement. That's because when your primary muscles fail you the body marshals a compensatory response with muscles not intended to bear the load, all of which results in the short-term effect of creating a greater risk of ensuing injury.

Why did we ever think that stretching protected us during a workout? Beside seeming intuitive that stretching gives you farther to go before pulling a muscle—an unproven assumption and not an especially common cause of injuries as it turns out—studies had shown a relationship between pre-workout stretching and fewer injuries. But those studies weren't testing only stretching, they were testing warming up as well.

With what we now know, it is possible that the studies that showed the benefits of stretching before working out actually showed only the benefits of warming up. Stretching may just have gotten credit for reducing injuries just by being along for the ride with a brisk warm-up. That means if you really want to reduce your chance of injury, you're better off first getting warm, then doing an easy set of bench presses with an empty bar after having gently rolled your shoulders, than you are doing a cursory pulling of your elbow just before crawling under that 225 pound set of disks. None of this should dissuade you from stretching, mind you. Just that you should save the stretching for its own hour.

Stretching Is Its Own Workout

For too long stretching has been viewed as a comfortable spell of relaxation more than the grueling, teardown corrective that it is. Maybe the softy reputation for stretching has something to do with how it is packaged—how you tend to sit on a mat on the floor, with the lights low and the music soothing when you stretch. Maybe stretching is falsely seen as a relaxing workout because even the elderly can become limber. Even the term "stretching" seems to underestimate the experience of what it really is, which is the athletic training of flexibility. Whatever the reason, we do a disservice when we play down what it means to stretch.

Putting your body into the self-supported positions necessary to relengthen muscles is a job unto itself, worthy of an hour of its own, and if you are stiff enough going in, a couple of days spent nursing sore muscles. If held and executed with the presence of mind necessary to get at a precise nexus of shortened muscle, the simplest-seeming flexibility movements can leave you sweating, shaking, and exhausted in as little as 30 seconds. Stretching can cause some of the toughest people in the gym to bail out in the middle of a 45-second flexibility pose. Stretching can kick your booty far worse than the leg press; it can leave you walking funny for days and ruin your ability to go bang out those squats you had planned afterward.

Beginning yoga classes are a great example of the unexpected duress of flexibility training. Guys are known for being some of the first to quit many power yoga poses, even though the gentler sex in the room are handling them just fine, the competition is fetching, and the walls are lined with mirrors. The reason: Pushing a weight or running down the road are both merely amplifications of activities we spend our days doing, but target your flexibility, and you might as well be trying to learn the trapeze at the circus. It is novel and strange. All of which is why you are going to need

to give flexibility training respect and time that it deserves, which means giving yourself the permission to fail and keep trying. Try to approach it like a training program all its own, as an hour all its own with little or no workout afterward.

Pay Attention to How You Feel

You can turn your brain off when running, swimming, and even cycling, but to stretch, you will have to pay attention. Stretching is precise, and to isolate the precise spots in your body that are tight

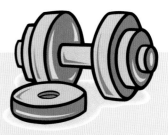

BE CAREFUL IN THE MORNING

You may want to hit the gym first thing in the morning, but if you have lower back problems, morning is a bad time to test the principle. There's a reason you tend to feel stiff in the morning. The intervertebral disks in your back become swelled with fluid during the night, limiting the range of motion of the lower spine. Bending in this state increases the chances you will transfer that compression by pushing a disk outward. If you do stretch in the morning and have lower back problems, bending should be done after an even longer period spent warming up, with greater sensitivity to the reality behind the stiffness. You aren't lazy, you're actually physically stiffer.

you often have to focus on the smallest changes in sensation and position. This is why, more than any other workout, flexibility training is about keeping yourself honest. Unlike weight lifting or running, the benchmarks of advancement in stretching are all highly individual. Only you know where in an extension you begin to feel tight and where you used to begin to feel tight. A stretch only is initiated, after all, between a self-perceived point of slight discomfort and a point just preceding (but never offering) pain. Sometimes the difference between a stretch and no stretch can be something as simple as the rotating of a limb, and in a matter of centimeters. This is why yoga instructors spend so much time prowling the floor and making infinitesimal adjustments to their clients' bodies. It's not so much that they are obsessed with precision (though that can be the case), as that they realize a stretch that doesn't make you groan a little might as well be time spent watching television. We can describe the stretches here, but you will only get a real stretch if every time you do it you think about how it feels. It's your hour, you're going to be back in the car or at the desk afterward. Why not pay attention?

Two Kinds of Stretches

You can stretch a muscle in one of two ways, either passively or actively. Passive stretching is what people think about when they think about stretching. It means using your own limbs, a towel, body weight, or the assistance of a partner to leverage and lengthen a muscle farther than its opposing muscle can do the job. When you prop your foot up against a telephone pole and

lean slightly forward to stretch your hamstring, for instance, you are passively leveraging your body weight against the resistance of the pole to lengthen the muscle. This may feel active, you took the step of lifting your leg after all, but in fact the force increase once you begin leveraging your hamstrings longer is passive—it has nothing to do with the ability of your quads to pull those hamstrings longer. Passive stretches also feel good.

Traditional stretching (even the non-western forms known as yoga) tends to lengthen muscles only passively. Thumb through any chart of stretches, yoga poses, or sequences and you will primarily see people sitting and leaning and pulling and being pulled by helpers to stretch a limb. "Maybe passive stretches were created as some sort of laboratory method to replicate something that happens in the field," says trainer Jay Blahnik with a laugh. "But a kicker doesn't have someone to pull his leg up for him."

As Blahnik and others have noted, there is much that is good about passive stretching, but it remains limited by one central fact: It has little to do with the practicalities of extending your range of motion. You aren't stretching your hamstrings to make them better at lengthening against phone poles. There is no sport that calls for such a stunt. You are stretching them to be longer when you need them when striding, which happens via the power of the quadriceps, lifting your leg far enough to do the work of stretching your hamstring.

All of this brings us to the second type of stretch, and one far less well known, which is an active stretch. To stretch a limb actively, you extend a limb farther than it is used to going, not through the use of a phone pole or towel or floor mat, but by the power of its opposing muscle. You basically move, lift, or extend yourself without outside help or forced leverage of any kind. The difference sounds academic, but in reality, passive stretching tests a skill that is not used in natural movement, and the active stretching tests a skill that is. Passive stretching is developed to the neglect of the partner muscle, and active stretching builds a muscle every time it stretches a muscle. Active stretching creates mobility, which is the only reason for stretching. It permits performance.

There is value to passive stretching; we sometimes fall and experience a muscle being passively pulled into a range of motion greater than it could have reached at the behest of its opposing muscle. You also reach a pleasurable state of relaxation from stretching muscles passively. But it's the active versions of most stretches that test the strength-flexibility relationship that constitutes real-world mobility. Your hamstring flexibility is of little use if you can't lift your leg with your quad far enough to be flexible. This is why Blahnik and others recommend that any stretch should be expressed actively first and passively second. In training to stretch actively, you may notice that you can't lift a limb nearly as far as you can leverage it, but over time, active stretching will minimize the difference.

How Long to Hold a Stretch

Studies show that a stretch held for 30 seconds helps flexibility more than one for 15 seconds, but that after 30 seconds, the gains made by holding your stretch longer are not as apparent. It won't hurt you to hold a stretch for a minute and a half, but chances are you will never need to do so in everyday life, and may not have the time to do so in everyday workouts. Power-yoga sequences dictate the duration of positions in terms of breaths, with 5 being the operative number in the case of the popular sequence known as the sun salutation. With controlled breathing generally coming out to around 6 seconds per breath, that works out to about 30 seconds in each position. Convenient, isn't it?

STRETCHING SELECTION

Like strength, you can approach stretching anatomically, working on your hamstrings and your pectoral minor, and get lost in all the body parts. Or, to make it more meaningful you can approach stretching, like strength, in terms of basic body movements. This makes the most sense. At the end of the day your flexibility is going to be expressed through your mobility, not your anatomy. To help keep you focused on function, the stretches described here highlight movements, as well as several active and passive ways to enhance mobility often impaired in athletes—movements related to stepping, rotating, bending, and extending.

Power Yoga

Traditional stretches exist for all the major muscles of the body, and while many are passive stretches, all are effective means to increasing your range of motion. One form of yoga, known generically as hatha yoga, is another way to target tight muscles. This is what most people used to think of when they thought of yoga—a series of poses, many seated, held to stretch muscles.

Pretty gentle and easy. You look like a pretzel. But that impression has been changing in the last few decades thanks to the popularity of the set of yoga sequences known as Ashtanga (also spelled Astanga). Compared to static stretches, Ashtanga yoga—or power yoga as Birch calls it—has more in common with sports performance, especially those sports that take place in the outdoors. The reason: Hatha yoga generally means holding static positions for extended periods of time—*passive* stretching, in other words. But the Ashtanga method (with its method of consciously maintaining a static contraction in the muscle opposing that which is being lengthened—*active* stretching in other words) strings its poses together in fluid movements and connects the progressions with deliberately paced breathing (one move takes place on the inhale and the next on the exhale, the next on the inhale). Moving, of course, is what happens in sport.

Moreover, where some forms of yoga often resemble contortionism, many of the Ashtanga positions are familiar to anyone who has ever done a push-up, lunge, or knee bend. By challenging you to move through positions in a controlled fashion, power yoga also develops your eccentric strength—the taxing of muscle in its elongated state and the kind of strength you need to decelerate quickly while coming down a trail. Because much of the workout is done on your feet, in multiple joint movements, and in all three planes of motion (front-to-back, side-to-side, and rotational) it is the definition of functional training—it builds the core while replicating linked movements you'll need in real-life situations. One-legged Ashtanga poses challenge your balance, and judging by research like that of a recent UC Davis study finding VO_2 max gains by yoga breathing, it even helps build endurance. By combining body-weight strength, flexibility, endurance, and balance all in one session, power yoga is quite possibly the perfect workout.

Surf legend Laird Hamilton says that thanks to Ashtanga yoga he's already seen improvements in his agility and his ability to extend into tough positions on the board. "The biggest thing it has done is given me more positions I can be powerful in," he says. "It's like your body is your tennis racket, and you're giving it a bigger sweet spot."

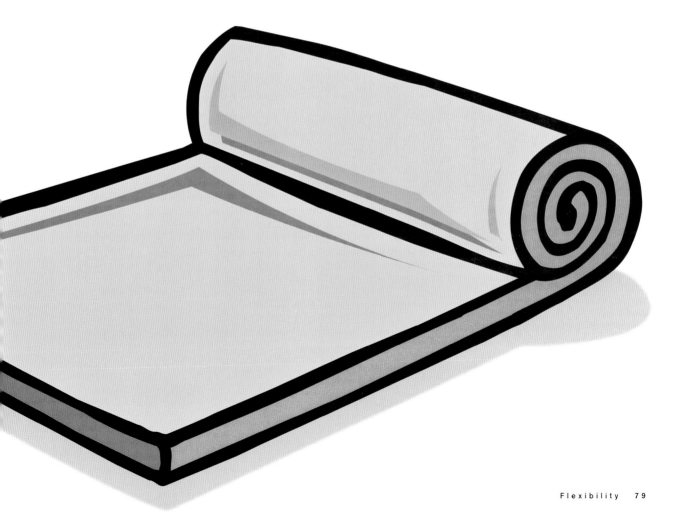

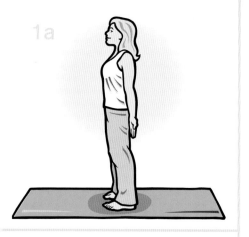

1a

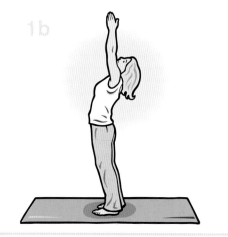

1b

Breathing

The whole point of power yoga is to maintain maximum flexibility in the ligaments and tendons, thereby giving the muscles more room to perform. That happens safest in the presence of heat. Most yoga methods devote a considerable portion of their lessons to the importance of modulated breathing. In power yoga, each carefully scripted change in movement is accompanied by either a controlled inhalation or an exhalation. The teaching advises you breathe in a specific pattern designed to pull the breath into the workload of the session. They call this form of breathing *ujjayi,* and it means breathing into your expanding belly, through your nose, with the back of your larynx closed. It's a snore, basically, and it generates heat throughout the body over time.

Sun Salutation A

If you only learn one stretch, make it the power yoga staple known as the sun salutation (SS). The SS is a nine-step series of linked movements that take your body through both active and passive stretches in the frontal plane. Your movements are also linked by your breaths and the breathing and step sequence become second nature after a handful of tries. You can repeat the series for as many repetitions as your form and strength allow.

The Sun Salutation is something of the rosary for yoga devotees—you can feel like you have repeated the series into a trance in some classes—but it does a lot of good with a small amount of work. Besides increasing both your forward-bending strength and flexibility through repeated forward bends and extensions, the series actively lengthens your spine via the power of your own reaches, and statically builds your upper body control, core strength, and pushing strength through cobra-like pushes and plank positions.

1. Start in a standing position, toes together, shoulders back, ankles apart, tailbone tucked under, and arms at your side. As with every power yoga breath, inhale deeply into your abdomen through your nose with your throat closed, lifting your arms above your head and pulling yourself upward from the crown of your head in a straight line.

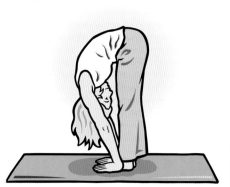

2

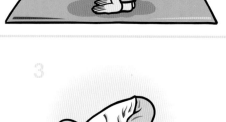

3

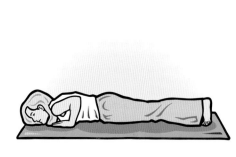

4

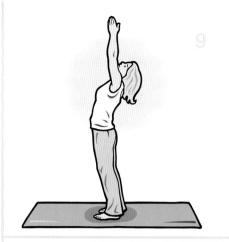

2. Keeping the lower back flat and abdominals contracted (think of the pulling of your perineum—the space between the anus and genetalia—upward), exhale, sweeping your arms downward, hinge forward at the hips to bring your palms to the floor. Most people struggle with the forward bend the most—it is the movement we lose first in our chair-bound society and in our excessively forward-stepping sports like running. It is also potentially risky for those with lower back pain. If so, bend your knees in order to bring your palms to the floor.

3. Inhale, extending your back straight to a 45-degree angle from your legs as you lift your head to look forward.

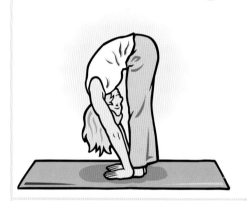

4. Exhale, placing your palms flat on the floor with fingers spread, and either walk or jump your feet back to a plank position with arms bent and your weight on your hands and your toes.

5. Inhale, dipping your chest and look up toward the ceiling arching your back into a position known as upward dog. (Those with back trouble can lessen the compression on the spine by resting their weight on their knees.)

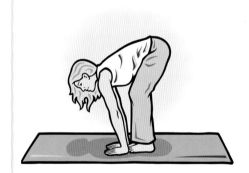

6. Exhale, turn your toes in, straighten your arms and lift your hips into an A-frame position known as the downward dog. Hold for five breaths, and watch as beads of sweat begin to drip from the tip of your nose.

7. Inhale, and hop or step to return to position 3.

8. Exhale, fold one last time into position 2.

9. Inhale, extending your spine upward and reaching with arms straight and palms together into position 1, before returning your hands to your sides.

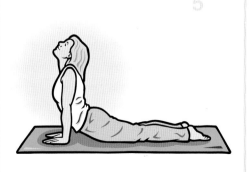

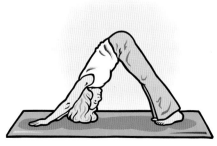

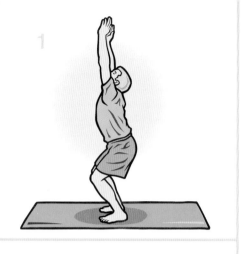

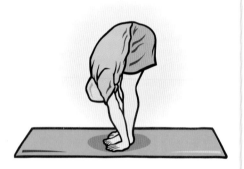

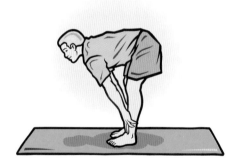

Sun Salutation B

This is an extended, 17-step version of the sun salutation, but one that begins and ends with a bent-knee reach and includes both right- and left-leg lunges out of the plank-upward dog-downward dog sequence. With two extra downward dog holds each totaling 5 breaths apiece (or 30 seconds, given the breath rate for abdominal breathing) the B-Salutation is both lengthier and capable of generating even more of the internal heat needed for your nerves to tolerate greater muscular lengthening. The starting pose builds bodyweight squatting strength. The lunges will build your lateral stability, stretch your hips, and build single-leg strength. Add to your session after the Sun Salutation A.

1. Start in a standing position, toes together, ankles apart and arms at your side. Inhale, bending your knees while lifting your arms above your head and pulling your torso upward from the crown of your head in a straight line.

2. Keeping the lower back flat and abdominals contracted, exhale, sweeping your arms downward and hinging forward at the hips to bring your palms to the floor. Bend knees if necessary, or if you have lower back problems.

3. Inhale, extending your back straight to a 45-degree angle from your legs as you lift your head to look forward.

4. Exhale, placing your palms flat on the floor with fingers spread and either walking or leaping your feet back to a plank position with elbows bent and your weight on your hands and your toes.

5. Inhale, dipping your chest and looking up toward the ceiling arching your back into upward dog.

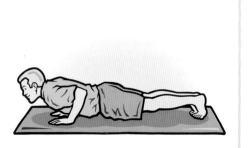

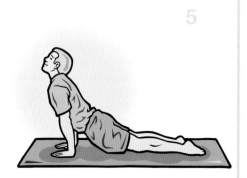

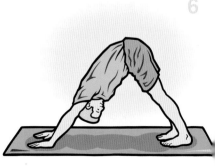

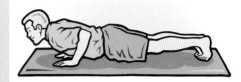

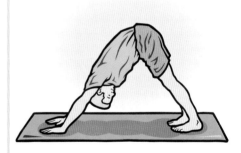

6. Exhale, turning your toes in, straightening your arms and lifting your hips into downward dog. Hold for 5 breaths.

7. Inhale, and with your left foot flat to the floor and angled slightly outward, step forward with your right foot into a lunge while reaching your arms straight above your head, into warrior pose.

8. Exhale, placing palms on floor and jump or step back to plank position.

9. Inhale into upward dog.

10. Exhale into downward dog, and hold for 5 breaths.

11. Inhale into a left-foot lunge with arms overhead into warrior position.

12. Exhale into plank, placing palms on floor and jump or step back to plank position.

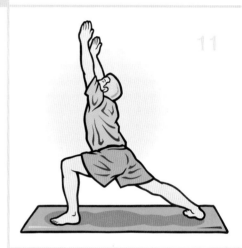

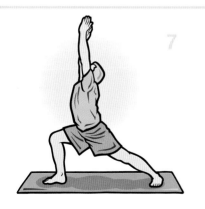

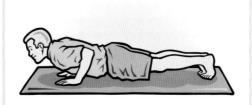

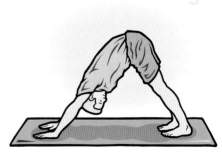

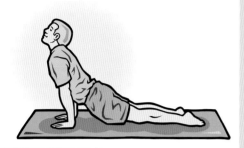

13

These are but a selection of the numerous active and passive stretches and yoga poses and sequences at your disposal in a flexibility training session. Over time you will become more aware of the particular areas of your body that have become tight and which deserve most of your attention, and you should feel free to structure your own flexibility session accordingly. Take the time to receive hands-on instruction in the form of a yoga class, as there is no substitute for individual attention when it comes to great form.

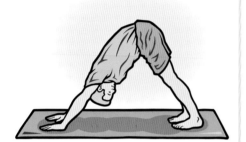

13. Inhale into upward dog.

14. Exhale into downward dog and hold for 5 breaths.

15. Inhale, hopping your feet to your hands to lift your chest and straighten your back.

16. Exhale, folding to bring your palms to floor (remember to bend your knees if necessary).

17. Inhale and stand to bent knees with arms overhead.

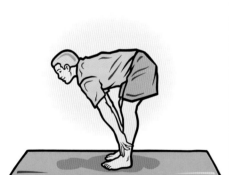

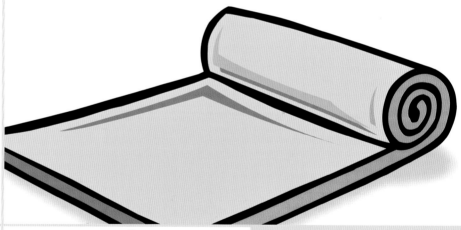

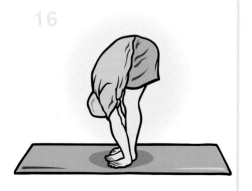

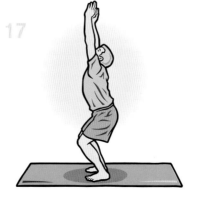

15

Active Back Stretch

Directions: From a standing position with knees slightly bent, reach around like you are hugging a tree, then bring your arms back to your sides.

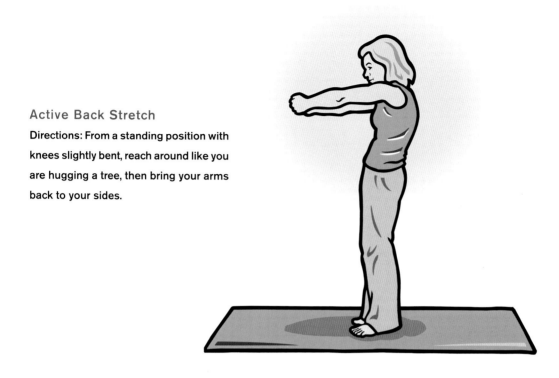

Active Hamstring Stretch

Directions: Lay on your back with knees bent and feet on the floor. Take turns lifting each leg toward the ceiling with its own quad strength.

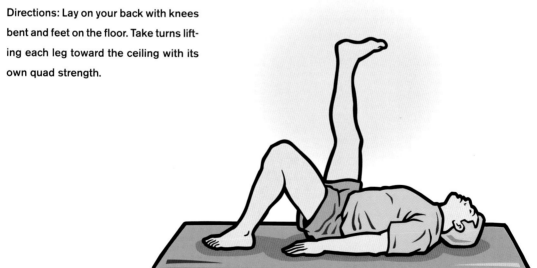

Passive Hamstring Stretch

Directions: Same as the active stretch, but finish by gently pulling your leg forward with your hands.

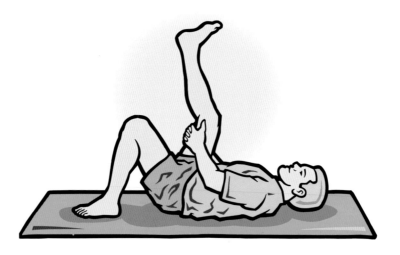

Triangle Pose

Directions: Standing with legs spread and hands at your hips, turn your right foot 90 degrees to point perpendicular to your body; turn your left foot slightly inward. Lift your left arm straight in the air as you bend sideways at the waist, descending so that your right fingers can grasp the big toe of your right foot or rest on the shin. Hold for 5 breaths. Repeat on the other side.

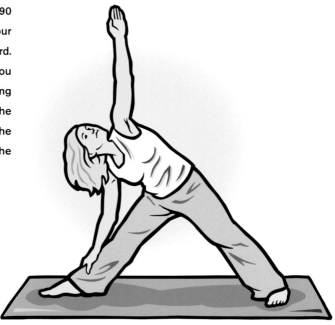

Extended Side-Angle Pose

Directions; From a spread-leg stance, turn your right foot 90 degrees to point perpendicular to your body and angle left foot slightly inward. Step into a lunge with right foot, and extend your left arm and torso in a straight vector crossing upward from your body at a 45-degree angle. Do not extend your knee past your toes. Hold for 5 breaths and repeat on other side.

Rotated Triangle Pose

Directions: Standing with your arms pointing outward with legs spread, right foot pointed perpendicular and left foot slightly inward, bring your left arm around so that your left palm plants to the floor on the *outside* of your right foot. Then, rotate your core and pelvis, turning your chest outward, so that your right arm points directly upward—or as close as possible. Hold for 5 breaths, using each exhale to slip deeper into the stretch. Repeat on other side.

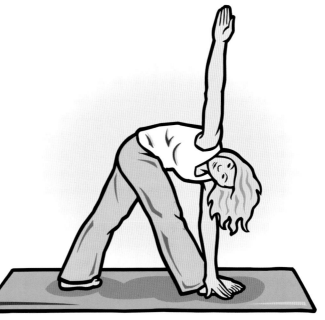

Active Calf Stretch

Directions: Seated with hands on the floor, back in natural alignment, and legs straight in front of you, flex to pull toes toward you and then release to point them outward.

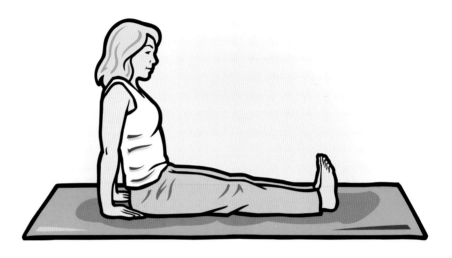

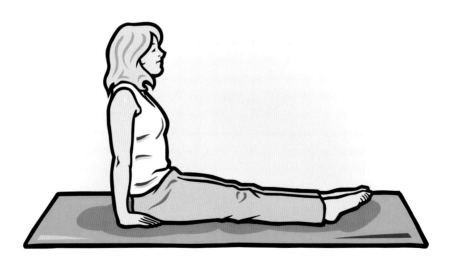

Active Glute Stretch

Directions: Lie on your back with arms at sides, cross your ankle over knee, lift other leg to 90 degrees, and rotate your foot in circles. Repeat with other leg.

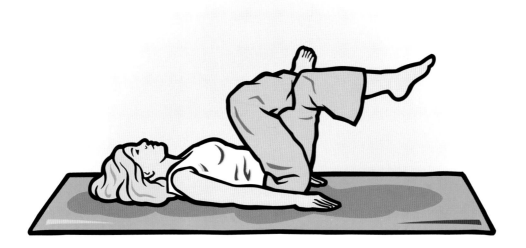

Active Quad Stretch

Directions: Stand and kick your foot toward your rear in a controlled movement, stabilizing yourself with your hands on a chair back if necessary. Passive finish: Lie on your side, reach back to grab your foot, pull toward your rear and hold. Repeat with other leg.

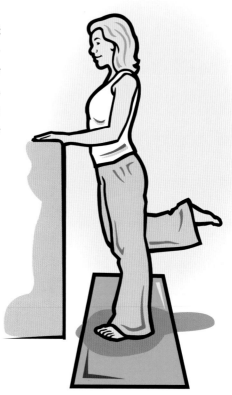

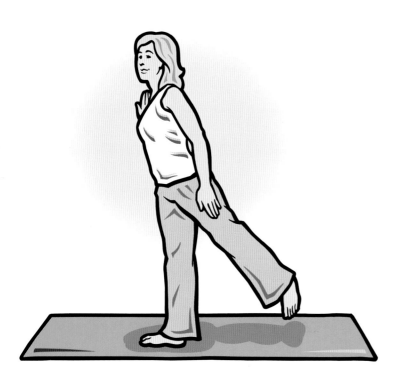

Active Hip Stretch

Directions: Stand, supporting your balance with a wall or chair if necessary, and swing your outside leg behind you in a controlled movement. Passive finish: Step forward with your supporting leg into a lunge, keeping your opposite leg extended behind and resting on the floor. Push your pelvis forward to stretch the hips. Repeat on other side.

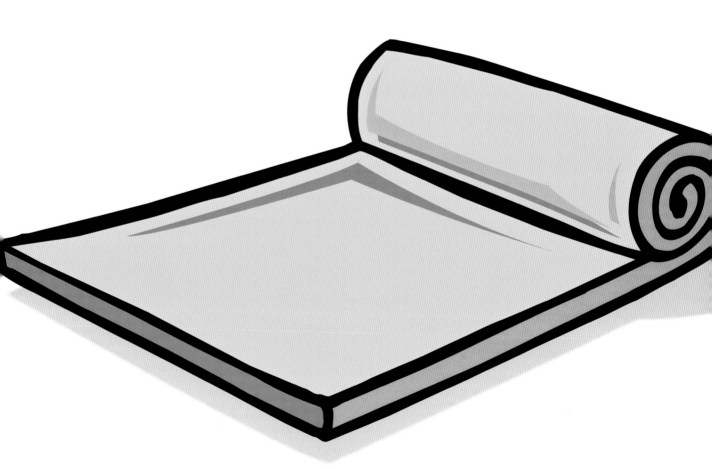

chapter 5
SPEED AND POWER

BY ADULTHOOD, MOST OF US ARE TOO SELF-CONSCIOUS

for the explosive workouts required to build speed and power.

ENDURANCE, STRENGTH, FLEXIBILITY—these are all very con-

trolled, very predictable, very sane. But power?

Power is for crazy bastards: short men in bar fights, entrants to lumberjack shows, dodgeball champs, and kilt-wearing, high-lander sport contest winners. After all, unless you have a score to settle with the bouncer or a hole to open off left tackle, why should you hop, leap, or toss medicine balls? And isn't speed strictly genetic? You can reach a healthy level of fitness and never put yourself through power training, a broad term that applies to the development of foot speed as well. But if you can find the time, it is a great way to expand upon a peri-od spent gaining maximum strength.

The world is filled with activities that demand more than the easy-listening tempo of jogging. Nearly every outdoor sport requires sudden bursts of first-step quickness at some point, and full-body propulsion. Outdoor activity can require power almost more than it does strength. Power, the term for force multiplied by dis-tance over time, is strength performed at speed. It describes your ability to gain extra

energy and recruit additional muscle when muscles flash-switch from recoiling to uncoiling. Academic? Hardly. Whether paddling, pedaling, climbing, or scram-bling, there will always come a time when you need to drop and spring. Maybe it's the

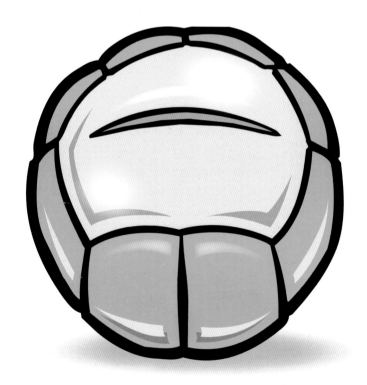

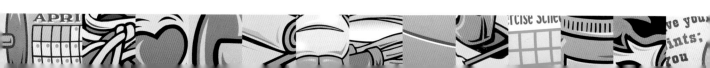

start of a triathlon, or a scrambling lunge to a hold just out of reach. Maybe it's a fast-approaching boulder one hard-stroke away from slicing open the hull of your kayak like a pistachio. Things can happen fast outdoors, and it helps to sometimes train fast if you want to be ready for them.

TRAIN SLOW, BE SLOW

That said, power training is sort of the spotted owl of the weight room. Most of what happens in the presence of the Please Wipe the Equipment signs is as glacial as a canasta tourney at the senior center. Chances are you curl barbells at a lazy cadence. Chances are your bench-pressing coordinates with the sluggish dirge of classic rock. All very understandable. The business of building strength is so disruptive to our comfort level, such an insult to our very cytoplasm, that slow is the only way to go in the beginning. The sensible clip of an everyday lifting pace ensures you are using correct form, avoids the cheat of momentum, and asks your muscles to feel both the raising and the lowering of weight for the greatest possible range of motion. And at the outset, this easy pace to ordinary strength training will build power in beginners. Ordinary squats, for example, can add as much as 20 percent to the vertical jump of the untrained. This happens because both power and regular lifting share the same zero-to-60 starting line, and everyday lifting of weights likely makes your muscles better at surmounting the first nanosecond of an explosive movement. As such, you can spend as much as six months in an ordinary weightlifting regimen while increasing power.

Although regular strength training will build your power initially, eventually it won't, and after that you won't derive power from the endless, everyday building of strength or simply by lifting weights fast. Power requires its own set of homework: medicine-ball throws, Olympic-style lifts (the various versions of the lift known as clean and press), and the unapologetically conspicuous jumping drills known as plyometrics, a needlessly fussy name for something as simple as jumping on boxes.

THE WINDUP FACTOR

The physiology of power is markedly different from that of strength, and as such, requires a whole new style of workload. Building strength requires overloading your muscle fibers to make them capable of moving heavier objects. Power, on the other hand, requires transforming the *elasticity* of your muscles, not to mention the responsiveness of certain spine-to-muscle nerve pathways. Both strength and power training are based upon the surprising fact that we actually produce more strength when we precede a movement with a quick countermovement, than when we pause to separate a launch from its windup.

It works like this: Any time you launch an object quickly through space, be it the weight of your body, bike, paddle, or a ball, physics and physiology require that you undertake two separate steps in quick succession. The first step is to put your muscles through a recoil-like countermovement, technically termed a muscular "stretch," for the way the muscle lengthens slightly at its ends when contracting in an eccentric (strength-slowing) fashion. The second step is to instantaneously throw your muscle fibers into reverse, quickly contracting to shorten them and extend your ankles, knees, hips, shoulders, or all of the above. Taken together, these movements are known in fitness parlance as the *stretch-shortening cycle* (SSC). The production of power lies in its briefest-possible execution, the tightest possible coupling between the recoil and the launch. Doing so literally gives the muscles more energy to work with.

But speed isn't all about muscle. Power has a neurological component. When you stretch a muscle quickly into a recoil, you momentarily possess greater strength via a spinal cord–mediated reflex. Thanks to your nerve pathways, you can enlist more muscle fibers into a power movement than you would otherwise have access to. Thanks to the power reflex and recoil, starting a jump from a sudden drop and launch will take you higher than from a stationary crouch. When it comes to making use of your elastic energy, it's use it or lose it; unless there is an immediate reversal from the stretching of your muscles to their shortening, this elastic energy will dissipate as heat. If you don't tie it to an explosive movement, the neurological benefit to a sudden countermovement all but disappears as well. As such, practicing a *fast* recoil-launch sequence is more important than practicing one that drops *deeper*. You need only to blink your eyes and miss the sight, as say, NBA point guard Allen Iverson bobs backward before reversing into an explosive drive forward to understand how a fast recoil can be brief to the point of immeasurability. This also makes the case for the fact that training power is less about how much weight you use as it is about how quickly you can use it.

THE BASICS OF POWER TRAINING

Classic power training involves three types of exercises: medicine ball throws, plyometric exercises, and Olympic style lifts. But unless you are trying to make the offensive line for the Cornhuskers, the Olympic lifts tilt the risk-reward relationship out of sync with general-purpose training. At the highest levels of power development you begin competing against endurance gains, and the lifts themselves are best approached through coaching. For that reason, the following workout focuses on the broad span of power development that can be brought about through jumping and throwing workouts. Your own body weight is often the only resistance you'll need to overcome.

Power Sets Run Short

To ensure that your body learns only a fast recoil-launch sequence (and it learns only what you experience in the form of practice), power training requires relatively brief sets. For best results, keep it to five to six repetitions with a medicine ball, and eight repetitions at most of a plyometric exercise set (for a total plyometric workout limit of 60 or so total foot touches).

Developing Pushing, Pulling, and Rotating Power

The best way to address pushing power in the arms and core is by tossing weighted medicine balls. For years these were made of leather, which reflected the fact that you were expected to do most of these drills with a partner. Provided you can find a concrete wall for the abuse of ballistic assault by medicine ball, the availability of durable rubber medicine balls in most gyms makes the solo medicine ball workout another option as well. Balls range in weight from 6–18 pounds; since working out with a ball that weighs too much will increase strength but not power, keep your ball to a weight you can chest pass 5–10 yards from a chair for six repetitions to a throw. Graduated medicine-ball progression moves from passing (two-handed outward), to tossing (two-handed upward), to throwing (two-handed overhead), and to swinging (side to side rotationally).

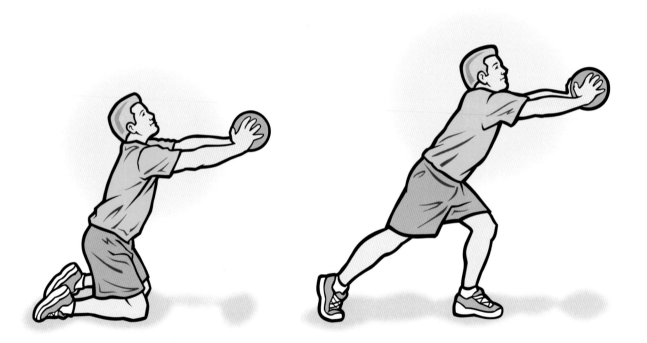

Medicine-Ball Chest Pass

Directions: Push the ball outward with both hands. If indoors, either stand or step into the throw. If outdoors, try doing so from a kneel—it allows full extension toward the grass—before standing.

Standing Scoop Throw

Directions: From a standing position, take the ball in both hands down between your knees, dip and reverse course, extending your knees and arms upward to throw the ball high in the air above you. Catch or let drop and repeat.

Dumbbell Horizontal Swing

Directions: Holding a dumbbell with both hands at arm's length in front of you, swing it to one side and back to the other in a controlled fashion, with your abdominals contracted and leading with your pelvis.

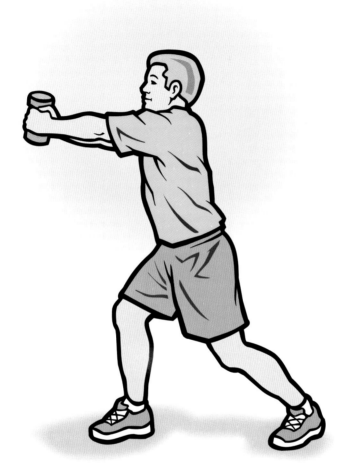

Plyometric Push-Up

Directions: Try doing push-ups from your knees with a clap in between. While these don't increase your strength over regular push-ups, they will teach the forward-pushing muscles of your upper body to recoil and push faster.

Developing Speed, Stepping, and Squatting Power

Plyometrics, or the practice of jump training, is as valuable to the business of sprinting as it is to the work of jumping. That's because speed is a lot more than just good genes. It's a common misperception that speed is genetic. While the ratio of fast- to slow-twitch muscle fibers given at birth may define an individual's maximum potential for speed, most of us are slower than we could be, not because of our age or lineage, but simply because we're rusty. "It's a muscle memory thing," says Donald Chu, Director of Performance Enhancement at Stanford and leading researcher in the field of plyometrics. "If you don't practice these skills they will desert you, leaving you vulnerable to Achilles, heel, and hamstring injury." There is a lot that makes a runner fast: a high strength to body-weight ratio, maximum anaerobic endurance, muscular stability, and a wide range of motion. But speed also comes down to something more technical: quickness in dropping and launching. Plyometrics is one of the best ways to prime your body for first-step quickness. By reducing your foot time on the ground, building more plyometric power is the ultimate precursor to speed.

Power training coach Jimmy Radcliffe says, "It teaches your muscles how to go from responding pliantly, like a tomato, to elastically, like a Super Ball." Both Radcliffe and Chu recommend starting your plyometric regimens with basic movements, then progressing to those with more complexity as you get more familiar. That means learning how to land before you jump, landing with your full foot, absorbing the momentum into your heel, knee, and hip, and keeping your back upright. The goal is to begin experiencing a measured reintroduction of your body to landing (drop and freeze), then jumping upward (a squat jump), then jumping *onto* something (two-legged box jumps), then forward hops, one-legged bounds, multiple versions of these, and finally, the plyometric apex that is landing and jumping put together (depth jumps).

To incorporate plyometric training into a regular workout, limit your jumps to once or twice a week, upward jumps to a height no higher than your hip and downward drops from a height no higher than your knee. For those weighing over 220 pounds, limit height drops to 18 inches. No one really benefits from dropping more than 43 inches—the work of absorbing the landing will slow you down too much to tag on a meaningful rebound. The majority of jumps can occur in a range of 12–36 inches, or a height that doesn't cause you to land your heels on the ground. To ensure quality of explosiveness, your jumps should start your workout. Find a dry, grassy area to place your box (if doing outdoors), or if the box is slip-resistant, a forgiving wood floor. You can use benches, stairs, or stumps as well. Wear shock-absorbent shoes. The less time your foot spends on the ground, the more explosive your legs become and the faster you get. It's best to keep all plyometric drills to 30 seconds at the most, for 60 touches per session or no more than 15 minutes in total length.

Drop and Freeze

Directions: Start your plyometric training by learning to stop a descent as quickly as possible with a drop and freeze. Starting on a box, bench, or stable object 18–36 inches off the ground, let your feet lightly step off the box. (Avoid jumping down off a box, it supplies force greater than your body will ever need to learn, and which your joints may not be able to accept.) "You want to drop or fall off," says Radcliffe, "so it's a surprise to your body." Land in a crouch stance, absorbing the momentum with your legs and then freeze in the position. "Try to stop the descent as quickly as possible," says Chu. "You are strengthening the phase that will eventually precede your takeoffs."

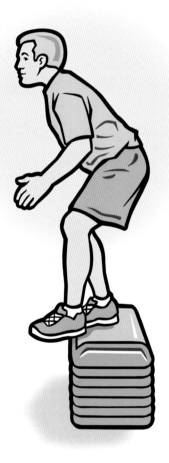
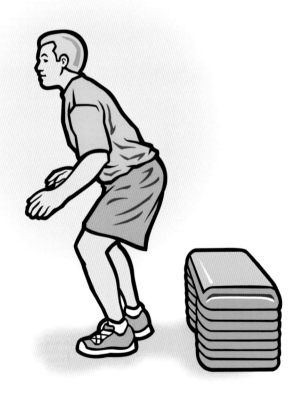

Two-Legged Box Jump

Directions: Stand in front of the box, crouch, swing your arms behind and then upward, springing yourself high enough so that you come down onto the box. Step down and repeat. "You want to shoot for as much hang time as possible," says Chu.

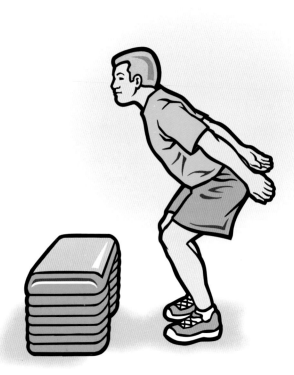

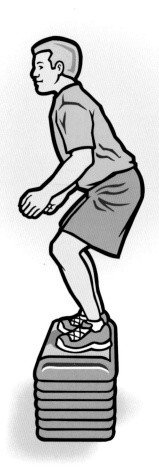

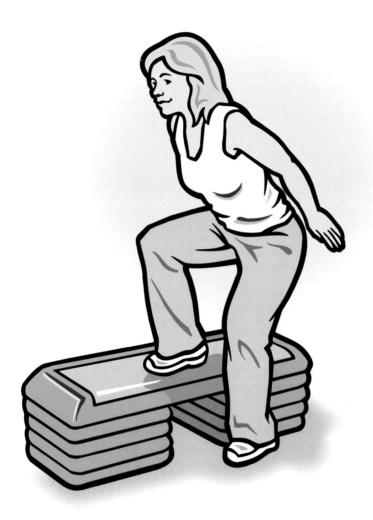

One-Legged Box Hop

Directions: Stand with one leg on the box and one on the ground, then drive your box-based leg in order to launch yourself above the box, landing with your feet in the same configuration. When reps are finished, repeat with other leg.

Stride Mechanics of Speed

At five foot eleven, former Buffalo Bills and Green Bay Packers receiver Don Beebe wouldn't have gotten nine years and a Super Bowl ring out of the NFL were it not for the fact of a blazing (4.3 seconds) 40-yard dash that held until late in his career. Instead of retiring to sell cars, he set up the House of Speed, a suburban Chicago-based clinic responsible for teaching the gift of Hermes to over 10,000 athletes in the last six years. "When I first started people thought you couldn't teach speed," he says. "What they should say is maybe you can't train world-class speed, but you can take someone with a 5 flat and make them a four-seven, a four-eight." (A tenth of a second, of course, is a lifetime in the span of a sprint.)

Besides exploding better off each foot touch, the average person can get faster by reworking some of the form problems that keep most of us from realizing our individual speed potential. It starts with this primary calculus: Speed = stride length X stride frequency. One way to maximize your stride length, is to make sure that when your leading thigh is extended, it is parallel to the ground. (For most of us at full stride, a Matchbox car placed on our thigh would roll onto the track.) To increase stride frequency, Beebe has athletes work on learning during each step to bring the stride leg down and beneath, rather than down in front, of their hips. "You want to rip the back of the striding knee towards the ground before it touches," he says. "Most people just lazily drop their foot straight down out in front of their hip, which causes you to land on your heel and then have to roll to the balls of your feet. That keeps the foot on the ground too long, which causes you to decelerate. You want to force it downward into the ground, both to generate more power, and to reduce the amount of time it's on the ground."

To make this adjustment to your form, he advises, start with a concerted walk drill, where you drive the knee and snap it down like a bear pawing at the ground. Move to a "funny run" practicing the same at 50 percent of effort, then build up to 60 and 70 percent efforts. "At 80 percent effort a lot of people start to lose the knee drive, " he says. It can take months to go from 50 percent to 100 percent, where if you watched your form in slow motion (a task highly recommended to those with a video camera) your form would look like Olympic sprinters. "Watch them in slow motion and you see how they snap their leg in front of their hip," says Beebe, "and how their swinging leg is always in front of their knee. I've seen athletes increase 1.5 to 2 tenths of second in form this way."

Top-End Speed

Finally, in addition to developing explosiveness and good form, speed depends on aerobic familiarity with working at your top end, both as a coordination issue and as an energy-supply issue. Building top-end speed requires pushing for speed under fatigue, then carefully notching away at the length of your rest intervals needed for recovery. You can do so, sometime in the later stages of a base-building aerobic training period by once a week making the effort to finish your runs or cycling sessions with two 30-second sprints, and, once your heart rate returns to normal, following each sprint with a light trot or cadence of no more than 60 percent of your ability, for 2½ minutes (or five times as long as the sprint). To improve even more, begin over time to reduce your recovery times in 15-second increments as you improve. Once your recovery time is down to 30 seconds between sprints, try to begin increasing the duration of your sprints.

Finally, keep in mind that while power training is a great way to add variety and intensity to your training year, each progression in complexity should come in its own time for your personal advancement. Chances are, after a few months spent lifting and running, your body may just be hungry for some landing, jumping, sprinting, and throwing. If so, work with that urge, and give your systems a taste of what it means to burn through fuel wastefully and explosively for a change.

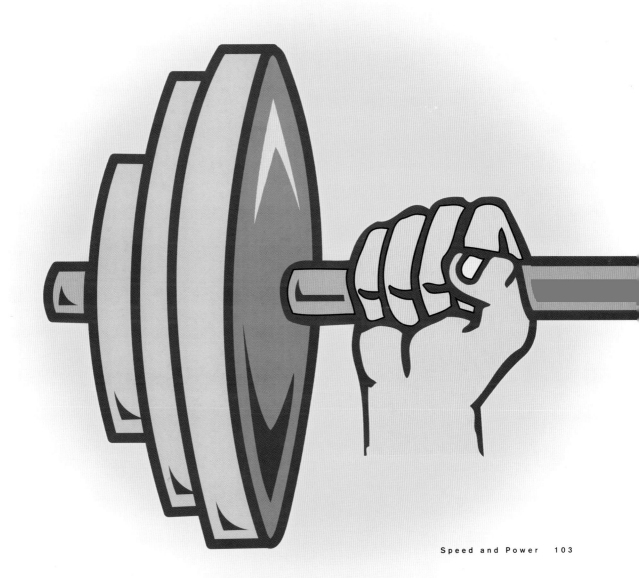

chapter 6
AGILITY

THE ESSENCE OF ATHLETICISM, agility is balance while in motion. Agility is something we admire in professional athletes yet hesitate to train in ourselves. **TYPICAL INDIVIDUAL TRAINING** comes down to running in a straight line for a very long time,

before heading off to the gym for a short spate of muscle building. You don't see too many grown-ups laying out their own private obstacle course on a Sunday morning in the park. We leave the shake-and-bake for Allen Iverson, the darting shuffle and crossover step for Derek Jeter. You have to be born with moves like that, we tell ourselves. Our feet would leave the station 10 minutes after our brain if we tried stunts like those. Right?

Not necessarily. Agility, or the ability to quickly change speed and direction in response to the unpredictable, is composed of a number of distinctly trainable elements. It's incorrect to assume that agility tends to be a skill you need specifically when a ball or team members are involved. You are hit with sudden surprises when you have objects flying and defenders attacking, and these surprises require you to change direction, momentum, and speed all on a moment's notice. You need agility to weave a soccer ball through a

thicket of opposing players, backpedal defensively in step with a wide receiver on an out pattern, or in step with a forward slashing toward the net, or to react quickly and accurately to the sudden crack of a bat or swing of a racket. Team sports clearly require agility, but there are elements of the unpredictable in solo and naturalistic activities as well. Trail running is largely an agility sport. Mountain biking is rife with sudden intrusions that require quick reflexes, as is road cycling, competitive or

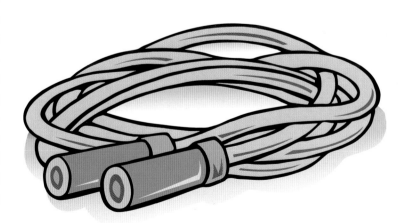

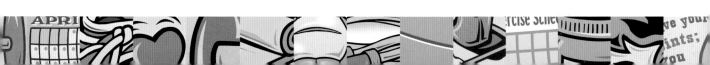

non, trail hiking, climbing, whitewater paddling, alpine sports, and nearly any activity that wanders off the predictable environs of a course somewhere. In its universality, agility represents the very best of athleticism: mobility, balance in motion, body awareness, coordination, and first-step quickness for both individual and team sports. You could say that agility represents the very best of human performance.

AGILITY PREVENTS INJURY

The primary reason for agility training however is preventive, as agility is key to reducing injury. It's no small accident that most knee operations result not from one-directional running, but from middle-aged and even younger athletes planting a leg to make a cut—on a soccer field, basketball court, baseball diamond, or ski slope—without the supporting musculature necessary to hold the integrity of the joint. Done correctly, agility training helps prepare you for those cuts by introducing your body to the forces created by sudden planting and pivoting, in a progressive and systematic format that reduces the risk of injury.

Most ankle injuries occur from landing on unstable surfaces—slippery rocks, mud, or another guy's foot while coming down with a rebound. They also occur through any attempts at descending without enough speed or foot control to keep your weight from shifting forward off your boot. "For outdoor sports, a lot of your training is going to be very linear," says Peter Twist, balance and agility trainer to NHL and NBA athletes and author of *Strength Ball Training*. "Running in a straight line, getting on an elliptical trainer or life cycle, are all very linear." But most of the situations you train for are multidirectional, with a lot of stops, starts, turns, pivots, and sudden changes in direction." Once we start to train exclusively linearly, we watch the erosion of the many bodily faculties required to do things needing agility, and the risk of rolling our ankles and turning our knees increases.

Fortunately, agility is like piano playing—it is a skill set encoded in muscle memory, and thus far more impervious to decay than, say, your lactate tolerance. What does that mean? If you take the time and build it progressively, you can sharpen your agility by as much as 30 percent. Once you do that, it will take a lot longer for your agility to erode than your gains in cardiovascular fitness.

THE BASICS OF AGILITY TRAINING

We all know that Barry Sanders looked unstoppable in his day—the way that he could teeter nearly sideways on one leg, right himself, and continue moving forward all at once. Bode Miller's phenomenal body control on the slopes has to be its nearest equivalent. But what exactly are their bodies doing? The raw skills of agility seem magical, but they are well defined and limited. These include:

- Backpedaling

- Transitioning into sprinting

- Making sudden turns and cuts with little loss of speed

- Foot control to execute fluttery shuffles, crossovers, and other lateral movements

◍ Flexibility and functional power for obstacle-surmounting maneuvers like hurdling and dipping

According to agility trainers Vern Gambetta and Steve Myrland, who are leading a lonely crusade to make training a smarter, more lighter-stepping practice, these moves all share five basic elements: body awareness, footwork, eccentric strength, coordination, and responsiveness.

Body Awareness

The most basic feature of agility is that of body awareness, or the awareness at the neurological level of the location of your limbs and trunk in relation to your center of gravity. At the end of the day you have to keep your hips over your feet, or gravity will take you down.

You hone body awareness through drills that make you disoriented. You can run, spin in a circle and continue on running; you can try different mat exercises you stopped doing when you were a kid (drills like tumbling, cartwheels, and reverse tumbles); you can put yourself through safer, precision whole-body movements such as bounding to your feet from a prone position on the ground. All of these drills will help develop your whole body awareness, and in turn body control.

Footwork

The second element to agility is a finely tuned control of your feet. This is the dancer's skill, and comes from having developed well-activated nerve pathways between your head and your limbs. Having a sense of rhythm helps you get foot flu-

ency, but almost any footwork pattern can be learned if you break it down into its smallest segments, then slow down those segments to a tempo you can do correctly (and almost any pattern can be learned if you slow it down enough). Training footwork also means learning to step lightly, or minimizing the amount of time your feet are on the ground. As Steve Myrland has noted, people often mistakenly believe you are supposed to go through an obstacle-course agility ladder with knees driving like pistons, when in fact your goal should be just the opposite. "You want your feet to be whisper quiet," he says, "barely leaving the ground."

Traditionally, you gain better footwork skill by doing ladder, dot, and other closed-space foot placement drills. These foot placement games help exercise and speed up the communication between your head and your feet, and a thorough approach simulates the most basic variations of controlled foot placement. These include: stepping forward, stepping sideways, shuffling sideways, crossover stepping, backpedaling, lateral weight shifting, and precise hopping movements like slalom jumping, 180 degree hops, and pattern runs through alignments of cones. The challenge in training yourself foot placement skills, is mostly logistical, to find ways to do this with low tech, ad-hoc supplies of the sort found in your natural surroundings.

Eccentric Strength

A third element to agility is eccentric strength, or the ability to slow your momentum with control. Eccentric contractions, you will remember, are those in which the muscle fibers extend slightly to slow or brake the forces against them. We may tend to assume that agility is about dashing your feet here and there, but put the skill under a microscope, as Gambetta has, and agility becomes something much more ordinary; stopping quickly. "I may be running on a trail and have to plant a foot to make a cut," says Gambetta. "To do that I have to have a strong eccentric contraction to reduce the force of my momentum. If I can't reduce force, I can't produce force."

The argument for specifically training your slowing muscle is even biological: Slowing movement is the opposite of stepping, even at the level of energy management. A recent study found that while climbing hills burned fat, descending hills burns carbohydrates. As such, you can't develop eccentric strength by pushing anything. The only way to train slowing muscle is to spend time slowing the movement of weight. Few of us ever do this. "An ability to reduce force is one of the biggest deficiencies I see at all levels," Gambetta says. We avoid eccentric training at our peril. "This is where you sprain ankles, tear your ACL, and pick up twisting injuries," he says. "You can't start if you can't stop."

In the gym you train the muscles to lengthen with strength every time you lower a weight slowly and with control. If you progress to an advanced level of basic strength, you can also build your eccentric capability by using so-called eccentric overload lifts, which ask you to take the unusual step of letting down slowly, in sets of 6 or so repetitions, 10 to 25 percent more weight than you can push up. (You do these either with the assistance of a partner in lifting the weight off you, or by yourself on a leg press by pushing out a weight with two legs, and lowering it slowly with one leg.) Because they occur at the joint where the muscle meets the tendon, eccentric contractions are a unique physiological demand. Training them can cause delayed onset muscle soreness (DOMS), a weight-training byproduct that lasts two weeks or more (see page 38). DOMS does not feel good.

Gambetta likes to build eccentric contractions first through simple body weight exercises like one-legged squats and basic box drops, then through amplification of body weight exercises. Once you find a partner, these include: lunging off a box raised marginally off the ground (4 inches or less); catching a medicine ball thrown from overhead while descending into a squat; and catching a medicine ball thrown from overhead while descending into a lunge. All of these should be done faster, if you want your body to be familiar with them when undertaking something faster.

Simply training yourself to stop from a run in the shortest amount of steps is another way to start up your eccentric strength. Try stopping a half-speed run in three steps. When that becomes comfortable, stop a three-quarter speed run in five steps. When you can do that, stop a full-speed run in seven steps.

Coordination

A fourth element to agility training is that ephemeral skill known as coordination, which means fluidity in moving numerous joints together in a unified movement. Coordination really becomes apparent when taking your first step in a sudden speed drill. The key to first-step quickness is simple—take your first step in the direction you want to go. This means not taking an unnecessary "dropped" step with the wrong foot or in the wrong direction before you get going. It also means not taking a first step that is too long (i.e., past the hips), thus causing you to spend extra energy pulling yourself up to the point where you can initiate a second step.

Some of us are born more coordinated than others, but simply training in movements rather than targeting muscles will assist in teaching your body's limbs and joints to work together. For this reason, coordination drills should employ multiple joints in succession whenever possible, especially when linked with secondary tasks like catching, throwing, dipping, or bending. Finally, certain body positioning helps promote coordination. You want to stay forward on your feet, and with your lower legs in positive (forward leaning) angles and under your hips. You want to take a shorter stride in the beginning of any speed drill. Revert to positions that allow immediate directional movement whenever possible. All of these principles promote efficiency, which is the heart of coordination, and can be trained through concerted footwork drills.

Responsiveness

The final element to all agility training is the ability to react to random stimuli. It is one thing to run an obstacle course that challenges your balance in motion, but true agility is only complete with an ability to change quickly without notice, as is generally required of all athleticism in a real-world setting. "I can do cone drills," says Gambetta, "but until I add a reaction component to it its not agility." The eccentric

muscles in your legs may learn to better slow your speed, your feet may know how to cross-over step without tripping and your legs may be coordinated at pushing off in triple-joint movements, but doing them in response to unpredictable stimuli will require activating the nerve pathways between your head and your legs.

You generally need a partner to train responsiveness skills. This means getting a friend to call out, tap you, or visually convey a sudden change in direction. It can be as simple as a friend 10 feet away dropping a tennis ball and asking you to get it on one bounce, or pointing to the left or right without warning as you sprint toward him. To train responsiveness on your own is difficult but not impossible (we can't exactly surprise ourselves with unexpected commands). The easiest way to train responsiveness on your own is purchase a cheap training aide, such as a reaction ball—a knobby ball that bounces in unpredictable directions. Drop it and chase it to catch it on one bounce, or you can also try just playing racquetball or handball by yourself.

PROGRESSION

The best way to train the components of agility is through progression. The most basic outline of this progression is speed, then complexity, then reaction. You want to start with basic movements at a slow pace, then progress into faster execution of basic skills, adding complexity as you go only when you master the previous skill, then linking multiple complex movements run at slow speeds and finally, adding an element of reaction to a fast, complex drill. You need to try the most basic skills at paces slow enough to do them correctly, because your body learns movements as code in your muscle, and if these are learned too fast to be undertaken correctly, your body will not be able to improvise on that code. Most of the time, that means that learning agility is a lot like signing up for your own personal dance classes, placing your feet in novel patterns, slowly and rhythmically. To use a different metaphor, applying progression to agility training is like learning a musical instrument, with your body as the piano. "You don't start out with "Flight of the Bumblebee" as Steve Myrland told me. You start out with "Mary Had a Little Lamb." Sometimes in learning the rhythm of a drill (and rhythm is entirely different from tempo), you may even have to count the steps out loud to yourself to learn a challenging footwork drill, says Myrland. But do so and eventually your feet will learn the movements well enough to pick up the pace.

BE CREATIVE WITH YOUR GEAR

Perhaps the biggest reason most of us avoid training agility is that it's sort of hard to do it on your own. Agility drills require not just forethought to draw out a course and then the humility to put yourself through the paces of some grassland soft-shoe, but quite simply, they generally require the sorts of gear that you would invest in only if you were a coach. We're talking about cones, hurdles, footwork ladders, dot drill mats, tubing, and explanatory videos.

Gear might be a primary reason we never train agility, but it doesn't have to be the decisive factor. You can replicate agility courses within a variety of basic settings using simple objects found in the outdoors or in your mudroom at home. If you live near a schoolyard you can use hash marks on a local football field for running drills. You can trace a basic ladder outline in a baseball diamond with a stick. You can use chalk to mark drills in soft blacktop. You can drop beanbags or baseball hats to mark a zigzag course and you can dart from boulder to boulder and back according to the command of a training partner. The drills that follow offer some ways to do this without a locker full of gear, either on your own or with a friend at your side.

THE DRILLS

Training for agility is best done on a soft surface where you can get traction, such as dry grass. Avoid doing agility drills on wooden floors, which can cause you to slip, or hard surfaces, such as concrete. Wear low-profile athletic shoes to limit your lateral instability. Few agility drills last more than 15 seconds at a run. Because they are fast and tax your creatine energy system, a system that is meant for only the very onset of a strenuous activity but which can resuppply itself with simple momentary rest, between drills rest around four times as long as you work, which in this case is generally a minute for each 15-second drill.

An agility workout can be as short as 10 minutes at the top of a regular workout or as long as 45 minutes dedicated entirely to agility, but the drills themselves should be short and in low sets, no more than 15 yards to a stretch, 5–6 repetitions on those that are repetitive and ending in 3 sets. "Agility should not be trained as an endurance skill," says Gambetta. "Trying to do too many reps without rest is teaching your body to learn a mistake, as it is no longer speed." You want to be sure to train agility early in a workout, in order to be fresh and alert. Because it is often eccentric in nature, which can cause unique muscular strain if done aggressively, limit your agility sessions to 20 to 45 minutes, 2–3 times a week.

Always warm up prior to an agility workout in a movement-specific pattern—with drills that resemble the movements you will be training, albeit at a slow and gentle pace. This could be slow circular runs, easy S-turns, shallow angles, or jog-ging through a line drill that has you planting and reversing directions.

Footwork, Body Awareness, and Coordination Drills

There is a basic progression to learning agility safely: Do simple, forward-footwork drills before doing side-to-side drills. Do side-to-side drills with simple crossover steps before advancing to multistep shuffles. Do these before learning to backpedal and then while changing directions. Practice stepping shuffles before trying their bounding and hopping versions.

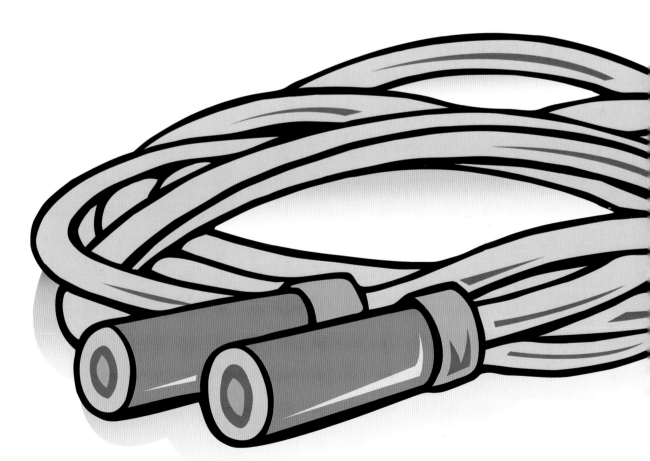

JUMPING ROPE

Jumping rope is an excellent way to develop not just upper-lower body coordination and cardio-vascular endurance, but foot control and foot speed. In the beginning it will be all you can do to string together a minute of jumping rope, but over time your coordination will increase to the point where you can do so at a brisk cadence for several minutes. Aim for a pace that allows 120–180 swings a minute or 2–3 jumps per second. The variations to jumping rope are as broad as your imagination, and learning several different jumps at the same cadence allows you to jump for longer and longer periods without getting bored and inviting trips that break your rhythm. Stay upward on the balls of your feet, be sure to flex your knees, jump as low as necessary to clear the rope and try to avoid looking at yourself in the mirror, as your brain will sometimes find the rhythm easier when the visual message is turned off.

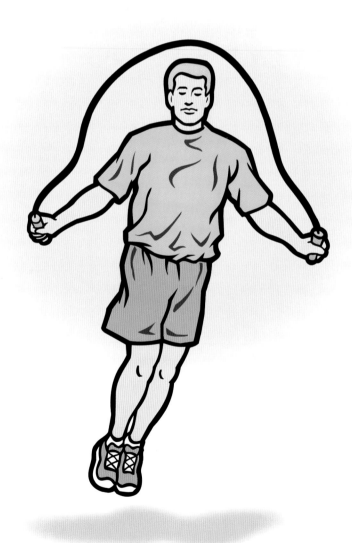

Here are five basic rope-jumping drills to get you started.

1. When you first pick up a rope, just get familiar with it through an easy double-leg hop at a cadence that gives you two jumps to each swing.

2. When this gets easy, start your jump rope sessions with double-leg jumps at one jump per swing, jumping just high enough to clear the rope, and taking care to reduce the sound of both your feet and the rope hitting the floor.

3. Progress to alternating single-leg jumps in a two-left, two-right cadence.

4. Move on to repeat single-leg jumps in sets of 10.

5. For a more plyometric rhythm that will help get you ready for ski season, try two-legged slalom hops to either side of a line in the floor.

More advanced moves include a crossover jump, where you cross your arms in front of you and uncross them as you bring the rope up from behind you, and two swings per jump.

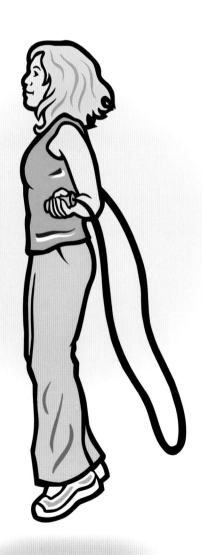

DOT DRILLS

For basic footwork speed there's nothing more basic than a dot drill, sort of a hopscotch for grown-ups. Etch in the dirt or draw with chalk on the blacktop a square just larger than shoulder-width, and mark it with five plate-sized circles, one in each corner and one in the middle. From here, you can create your own dot drills or you can try some basic ones, such as the following combination drill used by speed coach Don Beebe:

1. Skip from both feet on the lower two dots to both on the middle dot to both on the upper two dots, from front to back.

2. Next, start with both feet on the lower left dot, step your right foot to the middle dot, your left foot to the upper left, your right to the upper right and reverse the pattern to where you started at the bottom.

3. Next do the same but with just the left leg.

4. Then do the same with just the right leg.

5. Then do the entire drill from each corner with two feet together.

6. Next, start with feet spread apart, go to both in the middle then split them again at the top before jump-turning 180 degrees to your left so you can return facing forward, where you jump turn 180 degrees to your right.

Once you have mastered this quickly, do them in sets of six, and then string them all together and time yourself. It could take you a minute and a half to do them at your fastest, which is far longer than you will likely ever have to control your footwork so precisely in a natural setting.

Ladder Drills

Ladder drills can be broken down into three basic varieties, those moving forward, sideways, and backward down the length of the ladder. Forward drills offer basic movement control and rhythmic, forward weaving skills. Backward drills teach you how to pivot your hips while shuffling backward in a defensive movement. Lateral drills teach you how to move sideways with precision, building strength in the supporting structures of the knee and ankle.

With these three basic movements, however, you can compose an infinite number of variations of footwork patterns, from forward-stepping patterns to highly complex three-count shuffle- and cross-steps. Ladders can be purchased online from a variety of vendors (including www.performbetter.com), but they are basically a 10-yard span of 18-inch squares laid out in polyester webbing. It would be great to have your own ladder—they roll up conveniently and cost under $100—but it is not necessary. The primary goal of a ladder drill is to place your feet in predetermined spots (generally the length of a stride apart), not the precise configuration of that found in a ladder. With a stick or chalk you can mark one out on a dirt patch or blacktop, and you are on your way.

Try ladder drills slowly enough to do them right, then add speed once you have control. Lift your feet as little as you can, and drop down lightly on the forefeet. (The more time your feet spend in the air, the slower you are.) I learned the following drills from Myrland, who teaches them with Gambetta through videos and booklets available online. When you get bored with these drills, get creative and make up your own patterns—all that matters is that they are repeated enough to require you to force your feet to become more purposeful while being quick and light.

Forward Simple Ladder Drill

Directions: Alternating feet, step one foot in each box while moving forward as fast as you can do precisely. Next, step both feet in each box moving forward as fast as you can do with precision.

Forward Complex Ladder Drill

Directions: Starting with both feet to the left side of the ladder, cross your left foot into the first box, bring your right foot outside the right side of the ladder, bring the left foot to the right foot outside the ladder, then cross your right foot over to the next box and repeat. This trains you to cross your feet while changing directions suddenly, a cornerstone skill of agility.

Forward Plyometric Ladder Drill

Directions: Starting with your right foot in one box and your left outside, hop forward so that your left foot is in the next box and your right foot on the outside. Alternate in a slalom pattern down the ladder.

Sideways Simple Ladder Drill

Directions: Standing at its base and facing to the right of the ladder, cross your right foot over your left into the first square and then bring your left foot back into position in the following square down the length of the ladder. (This is also known as a half carioca.) Repeat with a left foot cross-step by facing the other direction.

Sideways Complex Ladder Drill

Directions: Facing the left of the ladder from a position to its right, lead with your right foot into the first square, bring your left foot into the same square and advance your right foot to the next square, follow with your left, return your right to the outside of the second square, then your left, and repeat.

Sideways Plyometric Ladder Drill

Directions: Facing to the left of the ladder with your right foot in the first box and your left foot below its base, turn 180 degrees to your right and land so that your left foot is in the second box and your right foot is still in the first box. Repeat in reverse down the length of the ladder. This skill is great for the sorts of coordinated 180-degree turns required of running moguls.

Backward Simple Ladder Drill

Directions: Standing at the top of the ladder on its left side and facing forward, step your right foot into the first box, bring your left foot into the same box, bring your right foot to its right outside and pivot your hops slightly to place your left foot in the next box, repeating the pattern as you descend. This teaches control in backpedaling defensively.

Backward Complex Ladder Drill

Directions: Standing at the top of the ladder on its left side and facing forward, cross your left foot into the first box, bring your right foot outside the right side of the ladder, return your left foot to its side, then cross your right foot over to the next box and repeat, turning your hips as you descend. This adds even greater complexity to backpedaling.

Backward Plyometric Ladder Drill

Directions: Standing at the top of the ladder facing forward with your right foot in the first box and your left foot outside, turn to the right 180 degrees to face down the ladder and land with your right foot in the next box and your left foot on the outside. Turn to the left and descend again, repeating as you go. Run the drill with your right foot in the box all the way down, and then run the whole drill using your left foot in the ladder.

First-Step Quickness and Eccentric Strength Drills

Prior to *starting* any cutting drills it is imperative that you learn how to *stop*. Failing to stop quickly while trying to change direction will keep your momentum moving forward while your foot is planted in place, potentially causing joint injury.

STOPPING DRILLS

One stopping drill is to run your half-speed pace and practice stopping in three paces. Then run your three-quarters speed pace and practice stopping at five paces. And finally, when this is easy, try running at full speed and stopping in seven paces.

The second way to build your stopping strength is through eccentric strength workouts. These include those bodyweight and assisted eccentric strength drills created by Vern Gambetta— lunges off a box then the same while catching a medicine ball thrown from above. If your basic strength is highly developed, you can undertake overload strength-training methods such as pushing a sled out with two legs and descending with one. Be warned, these can cause delayed onset muscle soreness, which lasts longer than customary muscle soreness.

Once you have practiced stopping at speed, you are ready to try changing direction.

LINE DRILLS

These are variations on the drills you practiced in middle school phys ed: Find a football field with hash marks. Starting at the goal line, run to the 5-yard line and touch the line, return to the goal line and touch, repeat to the 10, the 15, and the 20. You can also start at the 5-yard line, dash to the 10, return to the goal line and finish with a sprint back to the 5, touching the lines as you go. Last but not least, try to train some line runs that require you to run backward for 5 to 10 yards at a stretch, and add in 180-degree spins in the middle of the backpedal to finish it at speed with a forward run, which challenges your body awareness.

CLOCK DRILLS

This takes the eccentric and first-step quickness gains in the previous drill and adds a multidirectional element. Plot out a circle roughly 10 yards in diameter. Identify markers for every number on the clock face, and starting from the center, sprint 5 yards to the one, return to the center and repeat to hit each number until you have returned to 12 o'clock. For a more advanced version that builds your full body flexibility and planting movements, touch the lines with your hand.

CONE DRILLS

Cone drills are any course you set up to help your body move from forward, backward, and laterally through zigzagging patterns that challenge your equilibrium in motion. You can use any objects to mark out your course, though by giving you a 2-foot clearance to sidestep, actual cones keep you more honest. Lay out your markers anywhere from 5 to 10 yards apart, and practice zigzagging. In your field running drills, Gambetta recommends adding turning runs before gentle vectors and easy angles before advancing to sharper angles. Make sure each feels comfortable at the easier pace before adding speed.

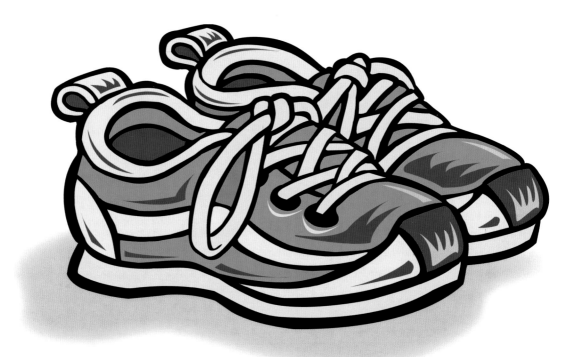

Responsiveness Drills

The final stage of complexity in agility runs is to add an element of responsiveness. Most responsiveness drills require help from a friend, as none of us can create our own circumstances of the unexpected, but nearly any of the drills above can be made to challenge your reaction skills with the simple addition of having a friend call out sudden changes in direction.

Here are some easy responsiveness drills:

- Have a friend hold two tennis balls outward, and drop one unexpectedly for you to catch at the first bounce from a distance of 5 to 10 feet away.

- From here you can progress to straight line runs toward the friend who then points out a command to cut and move to an angle when you get 5 yards away.

- Clock drills can be given a responsiveness component by having to hit numbers on the clock face when called out by a friend.

- Line drills can be interspersed with commands to stop and start.

- If you are without a training partner, use a reaction ball, which you can throw against a wall and be unaware which direction you will need to run to catch it on a bounce. Of course, the better you get, the harder you will be able to throw it and the farther you will be able to throw the ball from prior to catching it.

If you take the time to notice, agility training is more like playing than working out, and that should come as a welcome addition to your time spent in sweats. So much of training can feel like work, but in reality, most training is meant to enable play, and what better way to do that than by making up games to challenge your feet, limbs, and mind. It's hard to believe, given how enjoyable agility training can be, that it is one of the most responsible steps you can take to reduce injuries and increase your performance.

chapter 7
BALANCE

FOR BEING A SKILL WE ALL HAVE by the time we learn to walk, it's worth considering the breadth of balance. **BALANCE HELPS US IMPROVE PERFORMANCE AND CONFIDENCE,** as well as avoid injury, and we are capable of far more balance than we

have the occasion to develop. Stationary balance, the kind found in simply holding oneself upright with only imperceptible sway while positioned on an unstable surface, is capable of such variation from person to person that it is probably the only ordinary human skill we actually pay good money to see demonstrated in the company of lions and tigers and bears. As the high-wire work of those balance artists found in troupes such as the Cirque du Soleil would suggest, we may all have a Chevy for a balance system, but inside us lies the potential for that of a Porsche.

TRAINING STATIONARY BALANCE
Unless you work as a beam walker on a high-rise welding crew or a rig-worker on a sailing crew, you don't really have much need to refine your stationary balance system. So why train stationary balance? Stationary balance—as opposed to dynamic balance or agility—is the foundation to staying stable while in motion. If the prel-

ude to functional strength development is basic strength training, the prelude to agility is basic balance. Moreover, stationary balance provides the very foundation for identifying your strength deficits and postural imbalances, and is required to do the low-tech work of building muscle functionally.

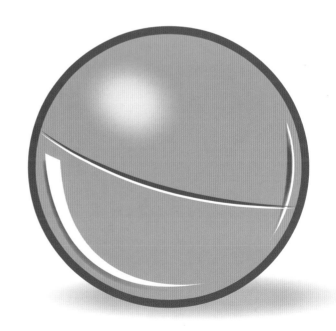

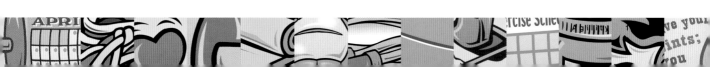

Let's face it, we lack standing skills. The simplest body-weight exercises often require far more stationary balance than most people possess. To do a one-legged body-weight squat, for instance, you need not only leg and hip strength, but the balance to hold yourself steady on one leg in the first place.

Undoing the deficits caused by how we live is another worthy reason to train stationary balance. Thanks to our sedentary, chairbound society, far too many of us need better balance, simply to enable everyday tasks like pulling on socks while standing on one leg, working safely on ladders, and stepping forward and reaching outward to pick up an object out of reach. Given that so many of the adjustments in muscular tension that create stationary balance are anchored in a strong abdominal core, and given that most traditional weight training artificially shores up your core with back supports and benches, even highly fit athletes can lack the ability to stay upright on unstable surfaces. So while it may entail time spent doing tasks like standing on one leg or using stability balls, foam rolls, and other gear reminiscent of a stay in post-surgical rehab, chances are you probably need to look at your stationary balance. There is nothing to lose and much to gain in spending a portion of your training year reacquainting your body with the vast network of muscles and nerve pathways that keep you from toppling while standing still.

The Physiology of Balance

When you move, your brain tells your body to move, your body does what it is told, and the brain moves on to something else, right? Actually, the body and brain are something of an arguing couple when it comes to movement commands. For every message the brain sends the body about where to place a limb, the conversation between your command center and your limbs has just begun, as an elaborate network of extracellular muscle-tension monitoring stations and stabilizing-movement initiators step into action. Once told by the brain to move a limb, the body sends back a confirmation message about where exactly the limb just went. The central nervous system compares any differences between the stated plan and the actual result, and if necessary, issues follow-up commands to stabilizer muscles needed to pull your body back over its center of gravity. This doesn't just happen when you are moving, standing on one leg or even a small platform such as a root, rock, or balance beam, it happens when you are standing still on two feet on the carpet at home. In monumentally small increments your body is always adjusting muscular tension to keep your sway minimized, and this feedback loop is a constant monitoring of your body's position in relation to its center of gravity.

Your body also continuously incorporates visual information to make postural changes necessary to prevent losing balance. Roof accidents, for example, are often blamed on visual blockages and other perceptual impediments to balance. The threats faced by guys who tear shingles for a living may sound inapplicable, but consider how it applies to climbing and hiking: At altitude, the body begins to sway both forward-backward and side-to-side, a sway increasing with each foot of distance between your eye and the closest object in its visual field. If there is no object to visually focus on within 15 feet, your sway is at its worst.

Seeing a tree move in the wind will also throw you off at altitude, as well as approaching an edge to a point closer than a 45-degree angle between your eye and the precipice. Such height-based anxiety will cause your core to tighten and your steps to become wider, both of which compromise your natural balancing micro-adjustments. Exhaustion will also be a factor at the physiological level in causing you to lose your balance. The more tired you are, the greater your body will sway in unstable circumstances and the less energy you will have to make sudden compensations to prevent a fall.

At the cellular level, the sensory elements of monitoring balance are also widespread. The brain-body hardware of balance derives from a disparate army of muscle and tendon-cell observers all sending data. They likely communicate through conduits long thought only to hold your body in place, the ligaments. What's this got to do with keeping you upright? Because all of these sensory messages happen below the level of awareness, running a loop from your muscles to your spinal cord and back, training for balance isn't so much about learning a set of rules as it is about exposing the body to unstable circumstances and making it figure out what to do to next. Making yourself unbalanced in this way forces you to experience the unconscious position-correction process enough that over time, your balance information super-highway becomes super-greased. Increase your exposure to instability and you have something much more useful than a mental experience with imbalance—you gain hardwired physical reflexes.

Progression

Research shows that athletes have better balance than non-athletes, but it also shows that strength training alone does little to improve your balance ability. One must train balance to develop balance, either intentionally or not, and to do so progressively. "Balance is developed by systematic exposure to a variety of unstable situations," says Bernard Petiot, training director for Cirque de Soleil. Progressively loading your balance isn't some arcane idea developed in a sports-medicine lab. Going easy before getting more complex is intuitive—all you have to do is observe the way today's street-sport athletes go about doing much the same thing with no coaching whatsoever. "If you look at Rollerbladers and skateboarders," says Petiot, "they will progressively increase the complexity of what they are doing. It's a key principle."

There are several ways to progress systematically in balance training. The most basic means is to start with floor exercises that challenge you with your very own body weight. These can include any sort of variation of standing on one leg, a task that can then be made progressively more complex by crossing your arms instead of using them like a high-wire pole, then through extending your arms in different directions, leaning forward, touching the ground, and pretty much doing anything with them while on one leg. To make any balance exercises harder, try closing your eyes. (Sight is a key tool in staying upright, and shutting it off heightens the work on your other bodily tools.) Having a partner then randomly nudge you this way or that while balancing yourself adds even more complexity to the skill, not least of which is the complex stability needed to respond to unforeseen forces working against your balance.)

Once you have grown tired of exercises designed to challenge your balance just with body weight, your balance training choices broaden substantially with the use of instability tools such as stability balls, foam rolls, wobble boards, and Bongo boards. Stability balls serve primarily to help strengthen your core, either through holding plank positions, or using them as a substitute whenever you would use a bench in the gym. The various instability boards and rolls are available for standing drills; just standing on these and holding a tuck position can add to your reflexes immeasurably.

The Drills

The drills that follow will guide you through the basics of what body weight and tool-assisted balance-training drills have to offer.

ONE-LEGGED HOLD ON FLOOR

Directions: Stand on one leg for 30 seconds, trying to keep your sway to a minimum. Repeat with the other leg. Increase your time to 1 minute, then progress as skill permits with your arms held outward, then while bending forward.

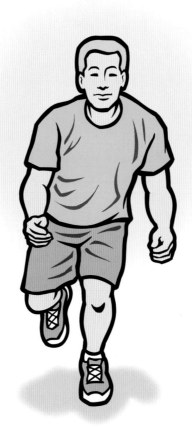

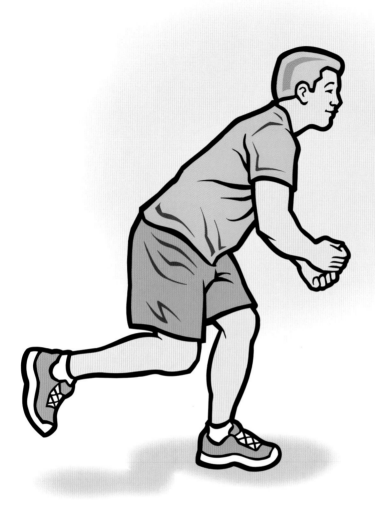

ONE-LEGGED FORWARD BOUND AND HOLD

Directions: Standing at a line, leap forward three feet with one leg and when you land on that leg, hold your position until you become stabilized. Repeat with the other leg.

ONE-LEGGED LATERAL BOUND AND HOLD

Directions: Standing on both legs, leap to the side a distance of three feet with one leg and when you land on that leg, hold your position until you become stabilized. Repeat with the other leg.

TWO-LEGGED DESTABILIZED HOLD

Directions: Stand with both legs on a foam roll for 30 seconds, reducing your sway as much as possible. Progress as your improvement warrants to a dynadisc, then standing on a wobble board, then on a wobble board in a slight crouch.

ONE-LEGGED DESTABILIZED HOLD

Directions: Stand with one leg on a foam roll for 30 seconds, reducing your sway as much as possible. Progress as your improvement warrants first to a dynadisc, then one-legged standing on a wobble board, then with knee in a slight crouch.

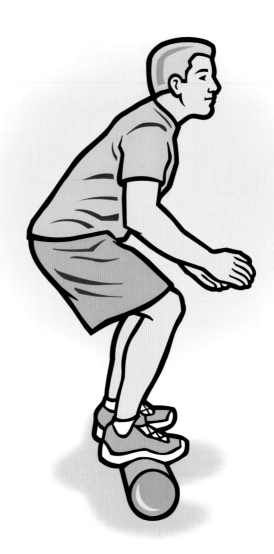

Two-Legged Destabilized Hold

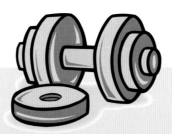

Like agility training, balance training is best undertaken in shorter doses that allow you fresh muscles and maximum mental alertness. Like agility, training balance will feel more like fun than work. Feel free to come up with your own derivations on exposing your system to instability—just make sure you proceed progressively and incrementally, and train in an area that will be forgiving if you lose your balance and go tumbling to the ground.

chapter 8
SPORT-SPECIFIC
TRAINING

TO GET GOOD AT SOMETHING specific, like paddling, biking, skiing, or climbing, it pays to move past the **GENERAL BASICS OF LIFTING AND RUNNING AND INTO ITS HYBRIDS**, the even smaller subcomponents of fitness otherwise known as sport-

specific training. Sport-specific training is the repetition of drills that mimic, hone, and sometimes overload ski-type movements for skiers, climbing-type movements for climbers, cycling-type movements for cyclists, and so on. The primary characteristic of a sport-specific training period, if you choose to take one up, is that after having increased your resistance and reduced the number of repetitions, sport-specific drills put that imperative in reverse, in order to build muscular endurance, rather than maximum strength. High repetitions—somewhere in the 20–30 range—are the general way to structure a sport-specific movement, and with relatively short breaks between sets, so as to not allow your muscles to fully recover. When taking up high repetitions, the resistance drops to perhaps only 60 percent of the heaviest amount of weight you could do once. The upside to reaching this stage of the training year is that you may find yourself finally feeling like your train-

ing is beginning to get tangible, to be applied in nature, and to look more like the sport you care about.

If you are a competitive athlete—someone who trains all year to wear a number on your back one day—you likely long for the stage of training where you get to leave behind the benches and start trying out movements that replicate your sport. But

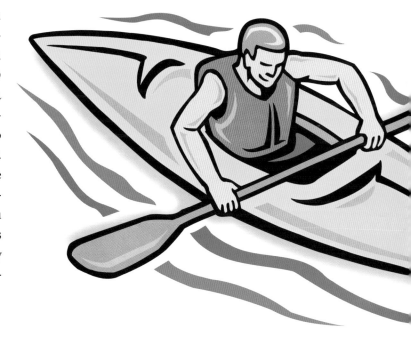

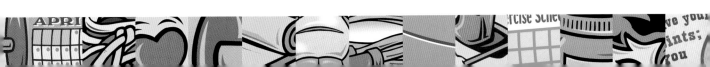

a lot of us aren't so competitive. Most of us never get to this stage of training, and that's not necessarily a bad thing. It's perfectly worthwhile to simply broaden your skill base in the widely practiced athletic categories like strength, flexibility, and endurance. If you can throw agility and power in there you are already steps ahead of most people not enrolled in an organized sport. But the best training is that which grows and changes throughout the year, and one of the best motivators for training has always been to increase your performance in a sport. To meet both of these goals, you ultimately benefit from moving from the general to the specific—to movements that closely mimic what you will be doing in your sport.

THE BASICS OF SPORT-SPECIFIC TRAINING

There are three key elements to sport-specific training: learning to observe your movements, perfecting your technique, and doing speed-specific workouts for your sport.

Observing Your Movements

The first step to sport-specific training starts with identifying the core elements of a given sport's movement. This means putting down your gear for a minute and taking stock of what you are actually doing that's making you sweat. Observing movements means developing the eye to see the rotational movements that link swimming, paddling, and throwing sports; the lateral weight shifting at the crux of both wall climbing and ski and skate sports; the forward-backward weight shifting of snowboarding, surfing, mountain biking, and windsurfing; and the lunging movements shared by telemark turns and traditional cross-country skiing. Once you identify the movements of your sport, all that remains is to train them in light but lengthy repetitions.

In other words, if you are into traditional cross-country skiing, the final training stage might add a two- to four-week period that focuses on building muscular endurance in the very step-lunging and poling movements you repeat while strapped into skis and boots. If it's skate skiing that you're practicing, you'll do better to train in movements that let you push off more laterally—say, by training with roller skis or skates. In the weeks just prior to getting down to paddling you might wish to incorporate a span of sessions dedicated to rotational drills designed to replicate the stroke you'll soon be repeating on water. To mimic the tottering of your boat, you can make the training even more transferable if you do it while seated on an unstable surface.

Alternatively, to ski downhill really well, a sport-specific training plan might reach a final tuck-endurance phase, where you spend some training time doing drills like holding your legs in a blue-run crouch for the duration of the longest run you want to be able to rip out on the real stuff. Or do the drills on balance boards.

Doing a sport itself is the only way to mimic 100 percent of what you need in a sport, which is why sport-specific movements can do only so much to make you better at your athletic calling. But what this last phase of preparation offers is a chance to break down your activity into its constituent elements, mini-movements that can then at times be loaded and repeated enough to give you greater muscular endurance not just with a muscle, but with a movement.

Technique

The precise execution of a given movement is too often overlooked by athletes in outdoor sports. There's something about the individualistic ethic of the forest, mountain, and stream that discourages slowing movements in order to fine-tune their execution. Most of this reticence is driven by the fear that tweaking our stride or stroke or pedal or posture is going to mean having to relearn how to crawl. Stay in a sport long enough, however, and you can't help but develop a grudging respect for good form. As fitness gains become smaller and the demands on training time greater, the idea of getting better by playing smarter seems like a good idea.

At the start of a sport-specific training period you might focus on muscle endurance and coordination, but prior to getting the timing right, it pays to slow down any movements necessary to enable you to tweak your form as well. "Culturally, people have bought into the idea that sports is about effort and hard work, to the exclusion of everything else," says swim coach Terry Laughlin. ". . . [But] The smartest thing any athlete can do is to improve their economy, and that's all about technique."

Speed-Specific Workouts

Gaining efficiency in a movement is fairly straightforward—you want to slow down and train the movement itself—but another way to increase your performance is to then do the reverse: train for these movements at the speeds, intensity levels, and durations that correspond to the energy system required of your sport. Soccer, for instance, requires lots of anaerobic bursts, while climbing often requires three-second tests of highly demanding levels of strength that rely on the creatine phosphate system. Neither of these would be sport-specific if you trained at an easy pace that was able to be fed by the aerobic (oxygen-fed) pathway. You would need to teach your body to tolerate repeated bursts of work interrupted by breaks— breaks which became shorter as your progress advanced.

THE DRILLS

The suggested exercises are but a short list of the many possibilities that exist for every sport. Use your imagination to come up with your own versions, and to ensure they be done fresh and at speeds that correspond to the work you encounter in your sport. Add them to your workouts at the start of each session, in sets of 25–30, or until your form decays, whichever comes first.

Kayaking and Canoeing

Crew-style rowing is a classic forward-backward pull stroke initiated in the legs, carried on further in the hips and finished with the pulling muscles of the back and arms. As such, it is an exclusively forward-backward movement, fairly symmetrical in the work it asks of the body, and fairly well covered as a lab task by most rowing machines. But the rotational and often pushing movements of sea kayaking, river paddling, and canoeing have more in common with the core-based work of wood chopping than they do with the movements honed on most rowing machines. As any kayaking coach will tell you, you can pull on the water with your arms, but your core has far more power and endurance.

The core is also vital to stabilizing you in the boat, and to transfer forces between your upper body and lower body, especially should you need to row the boat. The following drills will help you build a strong rotational and stabilizing core.

BALL-SEATED ROTATIONAL BAR PULL

Directions: Sitting on a stability ball, grab a fitness bar (preferably clipped onto tubing at both ends anchored to door knobs) with both hands. Rotate your pelvis to bring it down from your right shoulder to your left side, and from there, bring it up to your left shoulder and rotate your waist to bring it down to your right hip to mimic a paddle stroke.

BALL-SEATED CRUNCH

Directions: Sitting on a stability ball, walk your legs out and bend backward until your back slightly hyperextends, then pull your chin to your chest and lift the sternum just enough to crunch the abdominals.

FITNESS-BAR ROTATION

Holding a light bar over your shoulders with your abdominals contracted, your back straight, and knees slightly bent, with a controlled movement, rotate at the waist from side to side, leaving your trailing heel free to pivot with the movement.

BALL-SEATED TUBING ROW

Directions: Sitting on a stability ball, anchor a length of fitness tubing to a stable object in front of you. Pull the tubing in a row toward your sides. Or, hold tubing at side and rotate pelvis to row resistance.

Alpine Skiing

Staying crouched and leaning forward while skiing requires: muscular endurance in the legs and core; explosive side-to-side weight shifts; the hip mobility for 180-degree pelvic twists; the foot control and ankle strength to reign in a wayward boot resisting an icy skid; enough eccentric strength in the hips and thighs to slow your descent while carving turns; the balance to enable your legs to recover independently as they overtake separate obstacles; and the core strength necessary to buffer the extremely high gravitational forces being exerted on the legs.

And that's just for carving turns. Throw in some mogul hopping and you need dynamic explosiveness in the legs and hips, and even greater coordination between the stabilizing muscles required to anchor your midsection while in motion. In short, this is a sport that values very specific, highly unusual movements and body-control skills. With a little creativity, these movements can be trained in the gym and off-season.

STATIC SQUAT HOLD ON BALANCE BOARD

Directions: Standing on a balance board, carefully descend into a tuck position and try to hold yourself steady for as long as you can. When this gets easy, to add complexity, close your eyes, move your arms from side to side, or hold dumbbells.

TWO-LEGGED LATERAL JUMP

Directions: Working on a dry floor with sticky shoes with good cushioning, jump back and forth across a line in the floor that passes vertically between your legs.

TWO-LEGGED ROTATIONAL JUMP

Directions: Working on a dry wood floor with sticky shoes with good cushioning, jump from side to side over a vertical line, rotating your hips to land with feet together and pointing 45 degrees inward. Keep your jump height modest and your body in an alpine ski position (arms forward at your sides, ankles, knees, and hips flexed).

Telemarking

Telemarking, where the heel is free to come up off the ski and the skier controls his or her speed with interconnected single leg turns, is an increasingly popular form of alpine de-elevation. Compared to alpine skiing, telemarking asks an entirely different set of favors of your body. Instead of just moving down a mountain courtesy of boots that shore up the ankle and shin in 10 inches of polycarbonate, telemarking requires you to control your speed through a posture only weakly practiced in our daily lives—an extended stepping position. Telemarkers basically lunge their way down a hill, turn by turn, on the balls of their feet. To say the least, this is a sport that requires a deep skill base in the stepping movement so primary to human locomotion. It asks for enough single-leg strength to control the momentum of your entire body mass, and the body control required to keep your center of gravity over skis in even greater destabilization than is found in alpine skiing. When you consider that most people have a hard time just lunging their way around half of an indoor gym track, this becomes even more impressive. Sport-specific drills that get you ready for telemarking can emphasize power and control in stepping, especially in highly destabilized settings.

BACKWARD-STEPPING DUMBBELL LUNGE

Directions: Holding dumbbells or a barbell on your shoulders light enough to do repeatedly and with great control, step backward with one leg so that your weight rests on the ball of your back foot and the front leg descends into a 90-degree angle. (You can also do these by stepping forward, but the backward-stepping version is easier on the knees.) Return to the starting position and repeat from the other leg.

DOWNHILL TURNING LUNGE

Directions: On a low platform, turn your hips in 45 degrees to one side as you lunge downward. Step back up and repeat on the other leg, alternating directions. Go slow enough to drop with control, and hold yourself at the bottom of each step for a three count before pushing up into the next step.

STEP-HOPPING LUNGE

Directions: Step into a lunge, and then push off upward with enough force to cause your feet to leave the ground a few inches, landing in an upright position. Keep these sets short—the 8–10 range or until your form diminishes. Repeat.

Cross-Country Skiing

Cross-country skiing is primarily an aerobic sport requiring controlled lateral weight shifts. Because of the way it places you in a forward-leaning posture for an extended period, it requires exceptional muscular endurance in the lower back, hips, and legs. For traditional cross-country skiing, the kick is a calf and hamstring movement, while the stride is a lunge requiring both hip flexibility and endurance in the quadriceps. Cross-country skiing also requires repeated pulling motions generated in the arms and back and swinging movements initiated in the muscles of the shoulder.

BENT-OVER DUMBBELL SWING

Directions: Bend forward with your back flat, legs split forward and backward, and with a dumbbell in each hand take turns swinging them in controlled movements, extending your arm forward at a line with your body.

FORWARD LUNGE WITH BARBELL OR DUMBBELLS

Directions: With dumbbells or a barbell, step forward into a lunge and back, then repeat on the opposite side. Use a weight light enough to do high repetitions.

SPLIT-STANCE LEG DRILL

Directions: Standing with legs split front and back, and opposite arm forward and back, hop to stride in place, swinging your arms like ski poles.

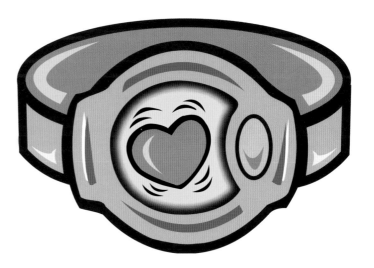

Skate-Skiing

While cross-country skiers stay in parallel, tightly coupled tracks, skate-skiers pole on every other push off of their legs, with their arms working in unison. As a stride with a side-to-side swaying movement, the key to skate-skiing is to never get stuck in the middle. You want your body fully committed in swaying from one side to the next with each push of your legs, with your head, shoulders, and hips all traveling in the same direction as your push.

SLIDE-BOARD DRILL WITH ARM SWINGS

Directions: On a slide board, step laterally into slides, and with every step to the right swing your arms to your right side, returning them above your left shoulder as you step to the left. These can also be done without a slide board, on a floor with shoes, simply stepping. (This can be undertaken from opposite side if you pole differently.)

LATERAL STEP-UP WITH BARBELL OR DUMBBELLS

Directions: With dumbbells at your sides or a barbell on your shoulder, step up onto a raised platform (12 inches or so) off to your side. Step back down carefully and repeat, then alternate sides when your reps are complete.

TWO-HANDED CABLE PULL

Directions: Pull a cable with both hands from a point above your right shoulder to your right hip, stepping to your right as you do so. Release it upward in a controlled fashion as you step back into position and repeat. (This can be undertaken from opposite side if you pole differently.)

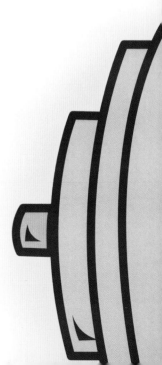

Snowboarding

The difference between the work of skiing and snowboarding is the difference between lateral (side-to-side) shifting of weight on skis, and the sagital (front-to-back) shifting of weight on snowboards. Both require a strong core and quad-hip complex, so you can benefit from squatting and lunging for both. But to replicate the snowboarding experience in the gym, start by thinking of lifts that emphasize fore-aft motions, and exercises that strengthen the abdominal core.

STABILITY-BALL BACK EXTENSION

Directions: Stabilizing your weight with your feet hooked under a stable bench or with legs spread and weight on toes, place your stomach and hips on the stability ball, cross your arms at the chest, and bend at the waist with a straight back as far as the ball lets you. Return to your starting position, careful to stop your extension when your body becomes straight.

DOUBLE-LEG FORWARD AND BACK HOP

Directions: Standing in front of a horizontal line on a soft floor with good shoes, bound forward a few inches with both feet and then bound backward, landing with knees bent. Repeat.

BALANCE-BOARD PARTIAL FORWARD BEND

Directions: Standing on a foam roll or balance board with knees bent, bend at the waist 45 degrees with your back flat and then straighten your back. Repeat.

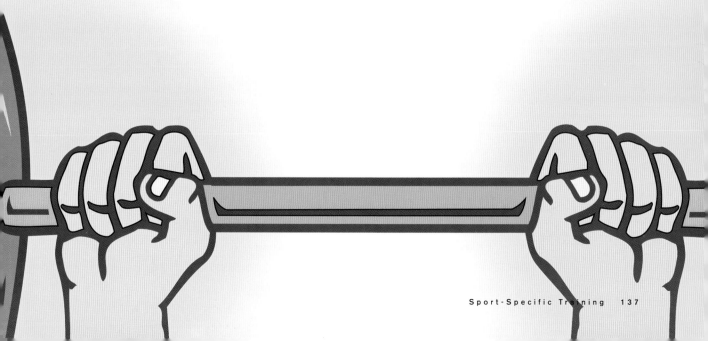

Climbing

Climbing requires hip flexibility, single-leg lateral stepping and squatting strength, grip strength, and pulling strength in the arms and back. Climbing works the arms far less than the legs, and much of the real work of climbing is in the ability to outlast long periods of muscular tension without getting a pump—the lactic acid overload that renders muscles temporarily useless. You can train for climbing by climbing routes on a wall, bouldering, and in the gym. Having a low body fat ratio is also extremely helpful for climbing, but given the importance of technique and skill, some great recreational climbers manage to get vertical without becoming overly trim.

PULL-UP

Directions: You can do chin-ups with your arms together and palms facing you, you can do pull-ups by turning your palms outward, or you can do wide-grip pull-ups by turning your palms outward and spreading your arms farther than shoulder-width. This offers a more functional variation of the pull-up, and one that places more of the work on your upper back.

WEIGHT-SHIFTING LATERAL STEP-UP

Directions: Standing next to a secure platform 12–18 inches high, step to the side with one leg in a smooth, committed weight shift, then push upward until you have straightened your outside leg, but with your exposed leg dangling. Step down in a controlled movement and when your repetitions are finished repeat on the other side.

WALL ROUTE

Directions: Pick a small route on a local climbing wall and do 10 laps.

IRON-DISK FINGER HOLD

Directions: Hold a heavy plate at your side—a 45-pound plate if possible but less if necessary with the fingers of one hand. Try to hold it for 30 seconds to a minute. Alternate sides. Build up your grip strength over time with longer durations.

Mountain Biking

Mountain biking requires many strengths: extensive eccentric muscular endurance in the upper body to absorb shocks during rugged descents, eccentric muscular endurance in the legs to slow the forces derived through the pedals, hamstring strength to pedal in continuous power output on the upstroke as well as the downward push of the pedal (see sidebar), leaping strength to launch your bike upward at the approach of a log or root, and lightning-quick hand-eye reflexes to dodge fast-approaching obstacles and narrow confines. Sport-specific mountain biking training can target shoulder stability, hamstring strength, pulling strength, and leg and hip power.

SINGLE-LEG PEDAL DRILL

Directions: Pedaling your bike in a safe area where you can be distracted with little risk of injury, stop and pedal in long stretches with just one pedal. Concentrate on keeping the uplift portion of the stroke a continuous link to the down stroke. Alternate sides and work until your legs get too tired. (See sidebar for another pedaling drill.)

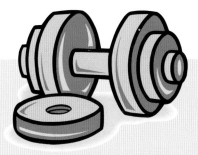

ROAD CYCLING LEG-PRESS DRILL

Much energy is wasted in a cycling cadence that veers either inward or outward. Women especially may find their knees wanting to angle slightly inward, due to their hip configuration. The following leg press drills teach your legs to pedal in a perfect vertical line from head to toe.

Two to three times a week for a period of three weeks, set the leg press at your body weight, and put one leg on the press. Making sure to center your knee visually over your second toe (it will probably want to veer over the big toe, or even veer so far as to be inside the line of your foot altogether), press the equivalent of your body weight one leg at a time in controlled, steady movements. From the front, you should be able to run a straight line from your hip joint to the middle of your knee to your second toe. Do these one leg at a time in 3 to 4 sets of 20–30 reps. Your goal is to teach your muscles the movement for endurance, not to build them. After three weeks, raise the weight and lower the reps, continuing to focus on form, but also now to work your climbing muscles.

STABILITY-BALL PUSH-UP

Directions: Place your hand on a stability ball with your feet on the floor and do as many push-ups as you can. Build up to 3 sets of 20 reps, then place your feet on a platform for added stability challenge.

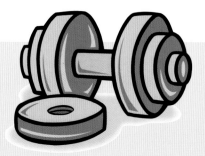

MOUNTAIN-BIKING FORM TRICKS AND EXERCISES

As a mountain biking coach, retired Olympian Ann Trombley spends most of her time hopping on her bike and having students follow her down the mountain. "If they can see the line I'm taking, they learn about picking routes and also get more courage that they can pull it off." Some of her general form pointers include going straight through the deepest part of a puddle rather than skirting its edge ("it's less slippery in there"), taking a line with the biggest rocks in it ("they aren't going anywhere"), and when it comes to single-track routes through the trees, knowing the width of your handlebars like the back of your hand. But her chief piece of form advice is on the subject of mashing, or pedaling just on the down stroke. To pedal better, you want each leg working all the time. "In order to climb hills with loose rocks you have to be really smooth. You can't be pounding. You want equal pressure all the way around."

"The truth is that Lance Armstrong was a bit of a masher in 1993 when he won the world championships," says Jeff Broker, biomechanist for the U. S. Olympic Committee. He says Armstrong did go on to develop circular pedaling skills. "It's not exactly central to being an all-around cyclist," he says. But mashers don't do well in loose soil, so in off-road cycling in particular you have to be a good peddler." While circular pedaling instruction places emphasis on the perception of pedaling even through the upstroke, the actual goal is far more humble—to get the foot out of the way of the movement towards an upstroke. To do so, you want to feel as if you are scraping mud off your shoe at the bottom of your down stroke, consciously unweighting the leg, then pulling it forward out of the upstroke. The best way to do this is to practice one-legged pedaling. One-legged drills work, because with one leg, the only way your pedal comes up to push down again is if you pull it. Trombley rests a foot on her water bottle cage for 30 seconds at a time, followed by one-minute rests, and then alternates feet. Doing pedaling drills at the end of workouts, helps as fatigue will produce the best results. Work up to a minute on, a minute off, alternating legs, for the last 20-minute ride home.

MEDICINE-BALL CATCH

Directions: Have a partner throw you a chest pass with a medicine ball, and in your catch concentrate on slowing the ball with your arms rather than catching it stiff-armed.

These are all possible ways to isolate and build sport-specific muscular endurance and technique, but they are simply improvisations, and you should feel free to think up your own. Provided you do not overload a movement too precipitously (the goal during sport-specific training isn't to build greater strength anyway), and provided you focus on simpler movements before progressing to complex movements, sport-specific training should be a largely intuitive process. Pick apart what you do in your sport, and find ways to build endurance at it primarily with your body weight and in the gym.

chapter 9

A 24-WEEK TRAINING PLAN

THE FOLLOWING IS A FLEXIBLE, six-month template outlining one way you can organize building your ENDURANCE AND STRENGTH over the course of four, six-week stages. In its complete form IT STRIVES TO ACCOMPLISH TWO THINGS: build

your aerobic endurance and progress your muscular training through four areas of strength—preparatory strength, basic strength, power, and sport-specific muscular endurance. The plan also includes sessions focused on flexibility, agility, and balance. This is a lengthy road, but keep in mind that if you choose to take it, everyone is different and you may need to modify a schedule to fit your own life. You should feel free to progress on a slower timetable than is listed here, limit your weekly days involved, or limit the number of weeks you progress down its path, should time constraints or your personal comfort level dictate a more limited level of participation. Think of this plan as a broad outline for integrating the many forms of fitness you have learned about so far in this book. As long as you progress systematically—building preparatory strength before basic strength before power, for example—you will increase your chances of success. Though they fall in the later stages of this particular plan, agility and balance workouts can be taken up at any time in a training plan.

Here's an overview of the training plan: The introductory endurance stage in the

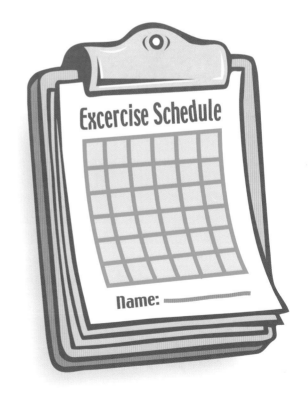

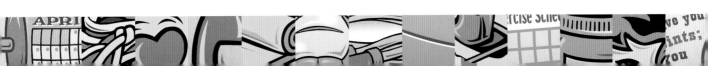

first six weeks is designed to set some running benchmarks and gradually get you up to running a half hour a day, five days a week. Your endurance workouts will then move toward some long, slow, distance runs in Stage Two (weeks 7–12), and then progress to runs punctuated with interval work in Stage Three (weeks 13–18), with the last stage (weeks 19–24) devoted to maintenance running and then a gradual taper in volume. The strength plan also begins in Stage One, with nine exercise categories designed to cover six primary movement patterns and their variations, as described in Chapter 3. During weeks 1–6 you want to build your tendons and support structures, so these exercises are performed at higher repetitions and thus at lower intensity, gradually increasing the number of suggested sets (1–2) if time and your body permits. During Stage Two, the strength plan reduces the total number of exercises to six, thereby allowing more sets (2–3), and at repetition counts that allow greater intensities (10–12). It is hoped that this approach will keep your time commitment manageable. By weeks 13–15, the plan offers some medicine ball and plyometric power-producing drills performed in numbers low enough to ensure they produce quality (6-repetition sets). The focus on strength wraps up in weeks 16–18 with a more carefree stint of agility training and balance drills, and in weeks 19–22 moves to sport-specific drills performed in numbers high enough to gain the local muscular endurance necessary to paddle, pedal, pull, or push your way through an enduring effort (20–30 repetitions per set). A brief taper is set in motion at the

end of Stage Four to set you up to be fresh and peaking at the end of six months. If you want to take part in a general fitness test of some sort—an active vacation—this would be a fine time to do so, before going easy for a few weeks and restarting and reformulating your next training plan anew. It is also possible you could use a general plan of this sort to prepare for a recreational sport season.

The plan contains a schedule with workouts Monday through Friday, but everyone's life is different, and some may prefer to train on weekends to leave a few more weekdays open. These days are merely a suggestion; as long as you get at least two days off per week and don't follow one hard running day with another, or schedule two strength days in a row, you can run or strength train when you wish. The idea is to get four to five endurance sessions and two to three strength sessions per week if possible. (If you ever feel especially worn out in any training plan, be it from a workout, life stress, or illness, it is better to skip days until you get your energy back than to work while exhausted.)

The run durations and lift repetitions are written as ranges—there's nothing magical about a precise number of repetitions, or minutes on the road—your body heeds general goals that progress over time, and your neighborhood running route might not wrap up in exactly 35 minutes, for example. In order to build daily running consistency, the workouts do end up double-booking your days with strength and endurance sessions at times. If this poses a time problem (each can take up to 45 minutes to an hour), you can run Monday, Wednesday, and Friday and strength train Tuesday and Thursday. An overall volume dip may make it take longer to see aerobic gains but the goal is consistency, and to do that you have to work within your own schedule. Avoid trying to push workouts into your days off in order to hit them all. Getting two dedicated days off is more important to your fitness than hitting every day on a workout chart. On days you take up both strength and aerobic workouts, the best order is to warm up first, then strength train, then run, to make sure your muscles are fresh for the complex work of strength training. To give your body a chance to recover within the larger schedule, weeks 4, 8, and 12 are lighter than those just before them. This is a principle to keep in mind when training—that you get stronger by easing up for a period at regular intervals. Again, ask your doctor before starting any workout, and cease any aerobic or resistance exercise if you ever feel pain, then get it checked out by a physician. Forget no pain, no gain; pain equals no gain.

Note: For all of the exercises in the plan, just the name of the exercise is given, and cross-referenced to its description and illustration in the corresponding chapters.

STAGE ONE: WEEKS 1–6

During the first six weeks of the plan the goals are: easing into regular running, getting dedicated flexibility time, setting endurance parameters, and building basic movement strength from two to three days a week.

Endurance

The primary goal of the first six weeks of endurance training is to acclimate your body to running four to five days a week consistently. The best way to do this is to measure your runs in minutes, not miles, run at an easy intensity level that elevates your heart rate but not so intense that you cannot converse while running. Warm up with 5–10 minutes of brisk walking and cool down with the same. It is best to not increase your duration more than 3–5 minutes at a time, once every two weeks. During your entire aerobic base-building period it pays to mix it up a little, by mixing in occasional harder efforts, sets of 3–5, 30–60-second interval sessions punctuated by rests of your choosing. These are known as *fartlek* sessions, a Danish word meaning "speed play." They are self-directed and can be undertaken after you are warm, and when you feel the readiness in your legs for some structured bursts—a quicker dash from this tree to that tree, for instance. The schedule also offers periodic tempo runs, a shorter run at a higher intensity of your choosing, but one sufficiently modest to enable you to keep the pace for the entire duration. The point is one of versatility: You want to build a base, but you also want your legs to become familiar with the biomechanics of swifter running early in any program. The chart on page 148 begins at 20–25 minutes for your first run; if 20 minutes is too much at the start, try two 10-minute sessions. The key is to begin at your fitness level in a flexible, sensible way.

ENDURANCE TESTS

During the start of an endurance training period many trainers recommend taking two simple self-tests to help you gauge the transformation of your aerobic capacity over time. You can do this by first measuring the heart rate at which your body begins to bog down from lactic acid accumulation (your so-called LT threshold pace), and then by measuring the time it takes you to run a mile at this heart rate. By comparing your pace at this same heart rate later in the program, you will have a better sense of your progress in aerobic conditioning.

Find Your Threshold Heart Rate

On a day you feel rested and well-hydrated, and after a gradual, 10-minute warm-up, strap on a heart rate monitor, then run the strongest pace you can sustain for 15–30 minutes. This pace should be harder than your conversational pace for your base-building work but not an all-out effort. If your monitor has an average heart rate function, at the end of this run check your monitor for the average heart rate for the period measured. If not, simply check your monitor every five or so minutes to estimate the average heart rate of the run. This rate is your lactate threshold pace, which you will need to write down for future interval sessions.

Find Your Threshold Mile Time

A few days later, or on a day when you are well rested and hydrated, run a mile at your threshold rate and write down how long it took. This will be the yardstick to gauge your increase in endurance at the end of the second and third stages of the schedule.

Strength

The goals during the first six weeks of a strength-training plan are to prepare your ligaments and tendons with modest weights and simple muscular endurance, identify basic stability deficiencies in the primary movements, and develop the core so that it may help reinforce your body for maximum strength and power training sessions to come later. Initially you can do this by lifting only one set of each exercise and by lifting light enough weight to be able to do at least 15–20 repetitions of each lift. Should a particular movement prove harder than others even at lower weights, that will give you a sense of those areas of your strength development that deserve more attention. Your body does much of its work in six basic movements as discussed in chapter 3. Cover these basic movements in the following nine exercises and you will begin to prepare your muscles to grow stronger in a balanced, functional manner. There are a host of possibilities for training strength in the basic movements, and the schedule here lists only three per movement; if you are experienced with others, feel free to substitute those.

NINE STRENGTH MOVEMENTS

Most of what we do comes down to a few basic movements: pushing and pulling with the arms, chest, shoulders, and back; stepping or squatting with your hips, rear, and legs; bending-extending at your waist and lower back; and rotating your pelvis.

The beginner, intermediate, and advanced strength training options that follow are designed to progress from working with body weight to working with instability, and finally to using loaded movements with dumbbells and if desired, barbells. Unfortunately, classifying the following lifts as beginner, intermediate, and advanced implies a superiority for some choices over others. In reality, the beginner options may be all you ever need, and indeed can deliver great gains in strength. Proceed with each lift only after a vigorous warm-up that leaves you sweating, and in the case of weighted lifts, with an unweighted set taken through its full range of motion. Between each exercise rest for 60–90 seconds or until your muscles feel refreshed. Choose a weight you can easily push 15–20 times. The goal is to familiarize your body with new movements.

Strength Movement 1: Squatting

Pick one:

Beginner: Leg press (page 44)

Intermediate: Dumbbell squat (page 45)

Advanced: Barbell squat (page 46)

Strength Movement 2: Bending and Extending

Pick one:

Beginner: Prone back extension ("Superman") (page 47)

Intermediate: Stability-ball back extension (page 48)

Advanced: Bent-knee dead lift with dumbbells (page 49)

Strength Movement 3: Forward Stepping

Pick one:

Beginner: Bodyweight lunge (page 50)

Intermediate: Dumbbell lunge (page 50)

Advanced: Barbell lunge (page 51)

Strength Movement 4: Rotating

Pick one:

Beginner: Oblique crunches (page 52)

Intermediate: Medicine ball rotation or lateral cable pull (page 52)

Advanced: Cable wood chop or reverse wood chop (page 53)

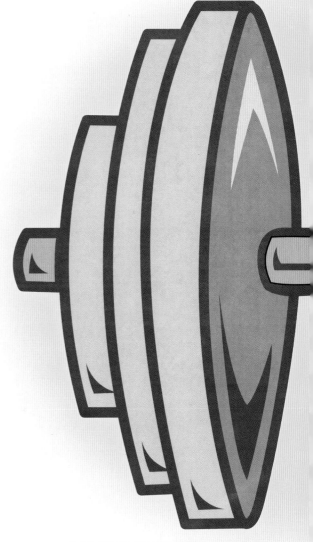

STAGE ONE	WEEK 1	WEEK 2	WEEK 3
MONDAY	20–25 minute run	20–25 minute run	Self test Find threshold heart rate
TUESDAY	Nine Strength Movements 15–20 reps 1 set	Nine Strength Movements 15–20 reps 1 set	Nine Strength Movements 1 set 1–2 sets
WEDNESDAY	20–25 minute run	20–25 minute run	20–30 minute with 5–10 minutes fartlek intervals
THURSDAY	Nine Strength Movements 15–20 reps 1 set	Nine Strength Movements 15–20 reps 1 set	Nine Strength Movements 15–20 reps 1–2 sets
FRIDAY	20–25 minute run	20–25 minute run	Self-test Find threshold mile time
SATURDAY	Flexibility	Flexibility	Flexibility
SUNDAY	Off	Off	Off

WEEK 4 (EASIER WEEK)	WEEK 5	WEEK 6
Nine Strength Movements 15–20 reps 1–2 sets 25–30 minute run	Nine Strength Movements 15–20 reps 1 set 30–35 minute run	Nine Strength Movements 15–20 reps 2–3 sets 30–35 minute run
Off	30–35 minute run	35 minute run
Nine Strength Movements 15–20 reps 1–2 sets 25–30 minute run	Nine Strength Movements 15–20 reps 1 set 30–35 minute run with 5–10 minutes fartlek intervals	Nine Strength Movements 15–20 reps 2–3 sets 30–35 minute run
Off	30–35 minute run	30–35 minute run
Nine Strength Movements 15–20 reps 1–2 sets 25–30 minute run	Nine Strength Movements 15–20 reps 1 set 30–35 minute run	Nine Strength Movements 15–20 reps 2–3 sets 30–35 minute run
Flexibility	Flexibility	Flexibility
Off	Off	Off

Strength Movement 5: Forward Pulling

Pick one:

Beginner: Incline pull-up (page 54)

Intermediate: Stability-ball dumbbell row (page 55)

Advanced: Dumbbell row (page 55)

Strength Movement 6: Overhead Pulling

Pick one:

Beginner: Lat pull-down (page 56)

Intermediate: Chin-up or incline chin-up (page 57)

Advanced: Pull-up (page 58)

Strength Movement 7: Forward Pushing

Pick one:

Beginner: Seated machine press or push-up (page 59)

Intermediate: Stability-ball chest press (page 60)

Advanced: Dumbbell or barbell bench press (page 61)

Strength Movement 8: Overhead Pushing

Pick one:

Beginner: Seated overhead machine press (page 62)

Intermediate: Stability-ball dumbbell press (page 63)

Advanced: Dumbbell press (page 64)

Strength Movement 9: Downward Pushing

Pick one:

Beginner: Tricep kickback (page 65)

Intermediate: Stability-ball tricep extension (page 66)

Advanced: Tricep extension (page 67)

Flexibility

You can train flexibility as many days as you have the time. What's important is to target a balanced approach to the movement that defines your sport. Often these are movements using legs and hips. Following is a list of suggested options, though the full range of stretches at your disposal is much broader.

- Sun Salutations A and B, 3–6 repetitions each (pages 80–84)
- Extended side angle and rotated triangle poses, 5 breaths each (page 87)
- Active and passive hamstring stretch, 30 seconds (pages 85–86)
- Active calf stretch, 30 seconds each side (page 88)

- Active glute stretch, 30 seconds each side (page 89)
- Active hip stretch, 30 seconds each side (page 90)
- Active quad stretch: 30 seconds each side (page 90)

STAGE TWO: WEEKS 7–12

The overall goals in weeks 7–12 are: more easy miles for endurance training, more intensity volume for basic movement strength training.

Endurance

In weeks 7–12 your endurance goal is to continue extending the duration of your aerobic base-building work, by gradually increasing the duration of your runs by 3 to 5 minutes every 2 weeks, with easier loads on the first part of weeks 8 and 12. Remember, the increases here are broad suggestions only; to prevent overuse injuries, it is important that you heed your own body's comfort level throughout any workout in deciding to increase your mileage. You should always feel free to reduce mileage or take days off if you feel under the weather or excessive soreness. At the end of week 12 is a good place, if you feel rested and well, to run a timed mile at your threshold heart rate to see how your endurance has improved. If your aerobic engine has become bigger, it will be faster than the timed mile you ran in week 3.

Strength

Your goals during this phase of strength training are to reduce the total numbers of exercises and repetitions per set, in order to free up your energy for overcoming a greater intensity of resistance relative to your personal limits. In order to build strength, you want to pick a resistance you can push 10–12 times, but maybe not 15–20 times. By reducing your exercises from 9 to 6, it will shorten your strength workout in order to accommodate more sets (which increases your total volume), and the increased time you might be logging during your runs at this time. As usual, these lifts have been chosen because of the way they require you to build your strength around 6 basic movements, rather than specific individual muscles.

SIX STRENGTH MOVEMENTS

The following is a shorter list of exercises in order to permit more sets within a given time frame, as well as to focus on those lifts where an increase in intensity is helpful.

Strength Movement 1: Squatting

Pick one:

Intermediate: Dumbbell squat (page 45)

Advanced: Barbell squat (page 46)

STAGE TWO	WEEK 7	WEEK 8 (EASIER WEEK)	WEEK 9
MONDAY	Six Strength Movements 10–12 reps 1–2 sets 20–25 minute tempo run at pace 10 beats below threshhold	Six Strength Movements 10–12 reps 1–2 sets 25–30 minute run	Six Strength Movements 10–12 reps 2–3 sets 40–45 minute run
TUESDAY	35–40 minute run	25–30 minute run	40–45 minute run
WEDNESDAY	Six Strength Movements 10–12 reps 1–2 sets 35–40 minute run	Six Strength Movements 10–12 reps 1–2 sets	Six Strength Movements 10–12 reps 2–3 sets 40–45 minute run
THURSDAY	35–40-minute run	35–40-minute run	35–40-minute run
FRIDAY	Six Strength Movements 10–12 reps 1–2 sets 35–40 minute run	Six Strength Movements 10–12 reps 1–2 sets 35–40 minute run	Six Strength Movements 10–12 reps 2–3 sets 40–45 minute run
SATURDAY	Flexibility	Flexibility	Flexibility
SUNDAY	Off	Off	Off

WEEK 10	WEEK 11	WEEK 12 (EASIER WEEK)
Six Strength Movements 10–12 reps 2–3 sets 40–45 minute run	Six Strength Movements 10–12 reps 1–2 sets 45–50 minute run	Six Strength Movements 10–12 reps 2–3 sets 35–40 minute run
25–30 minute tempo run	25–30 minute run	35–40 minute run
Six Strength Movements 10–12 reps 2–3 sets 40–45 minute run	Six Strength Movements 10–12 reps 1–2 sets 45–50 minute run with 10 minutes fartlek intervals	Six Strength Movements 10–12 reps 2–3 sets 40–45 minute run
Off	30–35 minute run	30–35 minute run
Six Strength Movements 10–12 reps 2–3 sets 40–45 minute run	Six Strength Movements 10–12 reps 1–2 sets 45–50 minute run	Six Strength Movements 10–12 reps 1–2 sets Self-test: Find your threshold mile time
Flexibility	Flexibility	Flexibility
Off	Off	Off

Strength Movement 2: Bending and Extending
Pick one:

Intermediate: Stability-ball back extension (page 48)

Advanced: Bent-knee dead lift with dumbbells (page 49)

Strength Movement 3: Downward Pushing
Pick one:

Intermediate: Tricep kickback (page 65)

Advanced: Tricep extension (page 67)

Strength Movement 4: Forward Pulling
Pick one:

Intermediate: Stability-ball dumbbell row (page 55)

Advanced: Dumbbell row (page 55)

Strength Movement 5: Forward Pushing
Pick one:

Intermediate: Stability-ball chest press (page 60)

Advanced: Dumbbell or barbell bench press (page 61)

Strength Movement 6: Overhead Pulling
Pick one:

Intermediate: Chin-up or incline chin-up (page 57)

Advanced: Pull-up (page 58)

Optional
Stability-ball crunches to failure

Flexibility
Same as Stage One. Feel free to mix and match other active and passive stretches and yoga poses of your choosing.

STAGE THREE: WEEKS 13–18

In weeks 13–18 the goals are: raising your lactic acid tolerance through twice-weekly interval runs, raising muscular power through twice-weekly power training sessions, and introducing agility and balance work.

Endurance

By this point you will have spent the better part of 3 months running almost every weekday at a conversational pace, interspersing your runs with periodic tempo runs and fartlek intervals, all while slowly building your duration so that you are running for as much as 45–50 minutes a day. What that means is that you have done your job as far as base building goes for the time being (remember, like strength, the sensible building of endurance is often a multiyear project). The running plans during this stage offer the option of alternating 5-minute intervals, 5–7 beats above and below your threshold heart rate. In running above and below your threshold heart rate like this, the combined average of the two types of work should be the equivalent of having you spend far more time at your threshold than it otherwise would tolerate, thus extending its ability to work aerobically. Over time you can extend these intervals as your fitness allows, for durations up to 10 minutes in length, and when that gets easier, you can shorten the rest interval just below your LT heart rate to half its previous duration, further adding to the effect of your body tolerating lactic buildup. The end of week 18 is a good time to retest how fast you can run a mile at threshold, to chart further improvement in your aerobic engine.

40-MINUTE INTERVAL SESSION

After a 12-minute warm-up at an aerobic pace, run 3, 3-minute sessions at 5–7 beats per minute above your threshold heart rate, each interspersed with 3, 3-minute sessions at 5–7 beats per minute below your threshold heart rate. Finish with 12 minutes of easy running.

40–50-MINUTE INTERVAL SESSION

After a 10 minute warm-up at an aerobic pace, run 3, 3–5-minute sessions at 5–7 beats per minute above your threshold heart rate, each interspersed with 3, 3–5-minute sessions at 5–7 beats per minute below your threshold heart rate. Finish with 10 minutes of easy running.

40–55-MINUTE INTERVAL SESSION

After a 10-minute warm-up at an aerobic pace, run 3, 5–10-minute sessions at 5–7 beats per minute above your threshold heart rate, each interspersed with 3, 3–5-minute sessions at 5–7 beats per minute below your threshold heart rate. Finish with 5 minutes of easy running.

RECOVERY RUN

This is a light jog to simply move your legs and speed recovery.

STAGE THREE	WEEK 13	WEEK 14	WEEK 15
MONDAY	Power Set 4–6 reps 1–2 sets	Power Set 4–6 reps 1–2 sets	Power Set 4–6 reps 2–3 sets
TUESDAY	40-minute interval run	40–50-minute interval run	40–50-minute interval run
WEDNESDAY	Power Set 4–6 reps 1–2 sets	Power Set 4–6 reps 1–2 sets	Power Set 4–6 reps 2–3 sets
THURSDAY	30-minute recovery run	30-minute recovery run	30-minute recovery run
FRIDAY	40-minute interval run	40–50-minute interval run	40–50-minute interval run
SATURDAY	Flexibility	Flexibility	Flexibility
SUNDAY	Off	Off	Off

WEEK 16	WEEK 17	WEEK 18
Agility Set 5–6 reps 2–3 sets	Agility Set 5–6 reps 1–2 sets	Agility Set 5–6 reps 2–3 sets
55-minute interval run	Balance Workout Reps held to good form erosion	Balance Workout Reps held to good form erosion
Agility Set 5–6 reps 2–3 sets	Agility Set 5–6 reps 1–2 sets	Agility Set 5–6 reps 2–3 sets
30-minute recovery run Flexibility	30-minute tempo run	30-minute recovery run
Agility Set 5–6 reps	Agility Set 5–6 reps	Agility Set 5–6 reps Self-test: Find your threshold mile time
Flexibility	Flexibility	Flexibility
Off	Off	Off

Strength

Since your body can optimally train only one energy system per training period, the increasing intensity of your endurance work and decreased daily volume present a good time to try out beginner and intermediate power training. Because power training taxes you differently than regular strength training, it is scheduled on alternate days to your runs. Be your own judge if you are ready, and if in doubt, proceed conservatively. As with all strength training be sure to warm up well before a power session. Proceed slowly with your first medicine ball throws to get the movement warmed up.

POWER SETS (can be done in any order)

Drop and freeze (page 99)

Two-legged box jump (page 100)

Medicine-ball chest pass (page 96)

One-legged box hop (page 101)

Plyometric push-up (page 97)

Standing scoop throw (page 96)

Dumbbell horizontal swing (page 97)

Practice sprint speed technique (page 102)

Agility and Balance

Agility and balance can be introduced any time during a training calendar, and indeed, much of the stabilization training that comes from balance work is most helpful early in a plan, to best point out areas where your body might be in need of more basic control. With so much of your earlier attention directed toward building basic strength and endurance however, agility and balance can be an especially welcome break from the intensity of power and speed development. Think of these as workouts for your nerves as much as your muscles. Agility sets listed here come in three skill levels. Move through them as your ease develops.

AGILITY SETS

Beginner

1. Jump rope for 5 minutes (page 112)
2. Dot drills (page 114)
3. Forward simple ladder drill (page 115)
4. Sideways simple ladder drill (page 115)
5. Backward simple ladder drill (page 116)
6. Half-speed run and stop in three steps (page 117)
7. Lunge off box (page 117)

Intermediate

1. Jump rope for 10 minutes (page 112)
2. Clock drills (page 117)
3. Forward complex ladder drill (page 115)
4. Sideways complex ladder drill (page 115)
5. Backward complex ladder drill (page 116)
6. Three-quarter-speed run and stop in 5 steps (page 117)
7. Cone drills (page 118)

Advanced

1. Jump rope for 15 minutes (page 112)
2. Line drills (page 117)
3. Forward plyometric ladder drill (page 115)
4. Sideways plyometric ladder drill (page 116)
5. Backward plyometric ladder drill (page 116)
6. Full speed run and stop in 7 steps (page 117)
7. Responsiveness drills (page 119)

BALANCE WORKOUT

1. One-legged hold on floor (page 124)
2. One-legged forward bound and hold (page 125)
3. One-legged lateral bound and hold (page 125)
4. Two-legged destabilized hold (page 126)
5. One-legged destabilized hold (page 126)

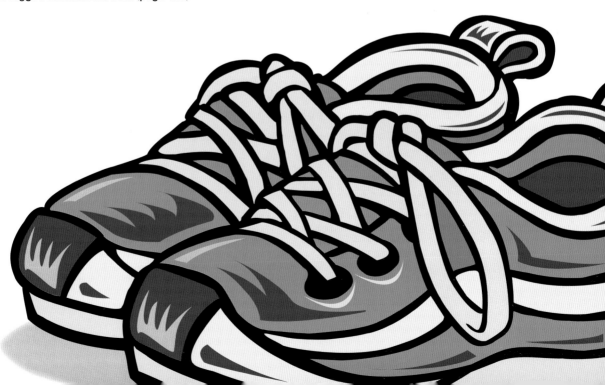

STAGE FOUR: WEEKS 19–24

During this last stage you will develop sport-specific muscular endurance, tapered endurance training, and peaking.

Endurance and Strength

You should not try to knock off a lengthy training plan without some sort of organized step-down in work any more than you should try to run your car for months on end without an oil change. In short, during the final stages of any lengthy period of training, the body benefits from working at some of your highest levels of intensity and abstraction down to some time spent working less intensely and more specifically. Stage Four is a great time to transfer to a few sport-specific drills done with low weights and in higher numbers, with the goal of making your muscles develop better endurance. Following are suggested drills for sport-specific training, or you can fashion your own drills around the movements you do in your sport, keeping them basic and mostly unloaded. Do them until your form is no longer good, or 20–30 times, whichever comes first. Following a brief sport-specific focus, your goal is to taper your overall workload in a gradual fashion for two weeks, to set you up for a period of peak-level training. Your strength and running plans are largely maintenance at this point. Doing either once a week is generally enough to keep your gains from eroding in the detraining process.

SPORT-SPECIFIC MOVEMENT SETS

Alpine Skiing Set

1. Static squat hold on balance board (page 133)
2. Two-legged lateral jump (page 133)
3. Two-legged rotational jump (page 133)

Telemark Skiing Set

1. Backward-stepping dumbbell lunge (page 134)
2. Downhill turning lunge (page 134)
3. Step-hopping lunge (page 134)

Snowboarding Set

1. Stability-ball back extension (page 137)
2. Double-leg forward and back hop (page 137)
3. Balance-board partial forward bend (page 137)

Cross-Country Skiing Set

1. Bent-over dumbbell swing (page 135)
2. Forward lunge with barbell or dumbbell (page 135)
3. Split-stance leg drill (page 135)

Kayaking Set

1. Ball-seated rotational bar pull (page 132)
2. Ball-seated crunch (page 132)
3. Fitness bar rotation (page 132)
4. Ball-seated tubing row (page 132)

Climbing Set

1. Pull-up/lat pull-down (page 138)
2. Weight-shifting lateral step-up (page 138)
3. Wall route (page 138)
4. Iron-disk finger hold (page 138)

REMEMBER, THESE ARE ONLY GUIDELINES, AND THERE'S ALWAYS NEXT YEAR

Make this workout serve you. Every workout is ultimately theoretical, and this general outline of how to work through a variety of training ideas in the course of your year is no different. While training is a great introduction to all of these methods and recommended, over a lifetime of training, you ultimately have to become your own coach, and that means being a person who will tell you to approach new work conservatively, try for more when you have it in you, and give yourself a break when your body is telling you something else.

STAGE FOUR	WEEK 19	WEEK 20	WEEK 21
MONDAY	Sport-Specific Movements 20–30 reps 1–2 sets 40–45-minute run	Sport-Specific Movements 20–30 reps 1–3 sets 40–45-minute run	Sport-Specific Movements 20–30 reps 2–4 sets 35–40-minute run
TUESDAY	40–45-minute run	40–45-minute run	Off
WEDNESDAY	Sport-Specific Movements 20–30 reps 1–2 sets 40–45-minute run	Sport-Specific Movements 20–30 reps 1–3 sets 40-minute run	Sport-Specific Movements 20–30 reps 2–4 sets 35–40-minute run
THURSDAY	40–45-minute run	40-minute run	Off
FRIDAY	Sport-Specific Movements 20–30 reps 1–2 sets 40–45-minute run	Sport-Specific Movements 20–30 reps 1–3 sets 40-minute run	Sport-Specific Movements 20–30 reps 2–4 sets 35–40-minute run
SATURDAY	Flexibility	Flexibility	Flexibility
SUNDAY	Off	Off	Off

WEEK 22	WEEK 23 (TAPERWEEK)	WEEK 24 (PEAKING)
Sport-Specific Movements 20–30 reps 1–2 sets 30–35-minute run	Off	Off
30-minute tempo run	30-minute run	30-minute run
Sport-Specific Movements 20–30 reps 1–2 sets	Off	Off
30-minute tempo run	30-minute run	Off
30–35-minute run	Off	Off
Flexibility	Flexibility	Flexibility
Off	Off	Off

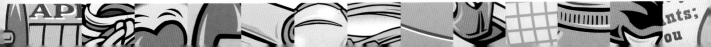

chapter 10
NUTRITION

IN SPITE OF WHAT THE FOOD POLICE MAY HAVE TOLD YOU,
good nutrition is neither a test of your virtue nor a memorization of your DAILY SERVINGS, CALORIES, AND GRAMS. Good
nutrition is taking up a conversation about how to STAY HEALTHY

in a society of cheap highly processed food. Whether your nutritional questions center around weight, modern food choices, or eating while training, the answers all tend to come down to how food works in your body and how we encounter food in the real world.

FOOD AND WEIGHT

The biggest reason so many of us even care about diet is because of the swelling desire, no pun intended, to do something about our waistlines. There are indeed good reasons to understand nutrition based on other concerns—such as the value of nutrition to sports performance, training, and recovery—that will be flushed out later in this chapter. But the first question we all tend to consider regarding nutrition stems from how to control our weight. This is a training book and not a diet book, but the subjects of weight and athletic performance do intersect.

Carrying extra weight is a hindrance to biomechanical efficiency, and one that will

adversely affect your aerobic efficiency as well. It simply takes more effort to move your legs when they are carrying more pounds. Extra weight also places added stress on your joints when undertaking repetitive, high-impact sports. You can, however, be overweight according to conventional standards and still be highly effec-

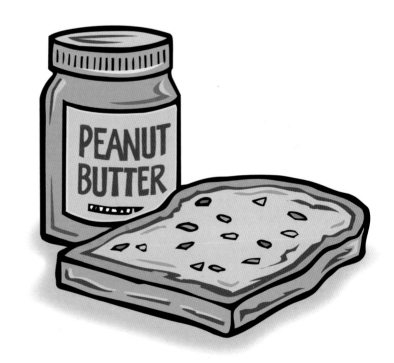

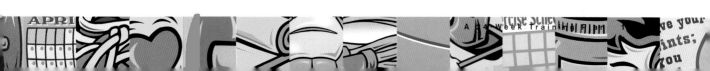

tive in many markers of fitness. Just take a look at the whoppers on sumo wrestlers and NFL linemen, athletes who possess extraordinary strength and power. Take in the soft-bellied builds of those extraordinarily flexible yoga practitioners who hail from the Indian subcontinent. I personally can attest to having watched a gentleman with an ass like a bear leave me in the dust during the Bar Harbor half-marathon. Of course, everyone left me in the dust on that sad morning, but that is another story.

While it may not be required for many tests of fitness, there remains a strong desire in this country to lose weight. Mostly we want to lose weight for better health and appearance. Appearance is subjective, so we will leave that little topic alone, but the endless push for weight loss as a health imperative is not as clear cut as the health authorities would have us believe.

Losing weight may make you gain weight. It may be your very efforts to lose weight that keep making you fatter. Most overweight people have lost and regained weight more than once. This happens through restricting calories, a method that ultimately leads to weight gain, not loss (more on that later). Moreover, weight regain after weight loss is potentially problematic for your health. Some believe it could well be that having lost and regained weight is what is raising our risk of diabetes, heart disease, and shortened life span, given the lack of attempts to take this factor into consideration in most studies linking obesity with poor health.

Weight and Health
Then there is the question of whether it is being fat that is dangerous, or whether the real problem lies in being sedentary. Studies linking obesity with health problems often overlook whether an overweight individual with poor health engages in regular activity. Whether or not researchers know it, there are many overweight people who live active lives, and when studied, some argue, they tend to fare little worse in terms of their health than do their thin and active counterparts. Indeed, the worst health outcomes tend to correlate with sedentary thin people. The fact that overweight people also tend to be sedentary may be what confuses our understanding of which factor, fat or low activity level, is the real disease risk.

There are some interesting arguments against body fat in relation to your health. Fat is a hormonally active tissue, for one, a substance that emits chemicals believed capable of causing the inflammation behind heart disease. Moreover, others argue that high caloric consumption creates more metabolic activity, spitting out more oxidative cellular structures, DNA-damaging particles that have negative consequences for aging and longevity.

But these are theories, at this point, and often based primarily on studies of mice and rats. Making the link from theories to the reality of disease in those who are fat is not as certain as we would like to believe, and thus there are better reasons to talk about nutrition in relation to weight than simply health. The best reasons to understand nutrition and weight are just three: It is desirable that normal-weight individuals limit the extent of future weight gain. It is desirable to lose weight, if one is to do so, in a way that will not promote weight regain. And it is desirable for athletes to eat in a way that facilitates training and recovery. For each of those goals, it is helpful to take a brief look at the fundamentals of food, and the short list of sensible findings you can take from the evolving research on nutrition.

NUTRITION 101

Your body eats just three different things. You could pick up a handful of dirt and put it in your mouth, but your body would send it right out the other end. Aside from vitamins, certain plant-derived phytochemicals, and minerals (some of which might be available in a handful of dirt, by the way), in all of creation there are only three essential compounds outside of air and water that your body requires to live. These are known meta-nutrients, and they are proteins, carbohydrates, and fats. You need all three (mostly carbohydrates, with protein and fats making up the difference) for energy, cell repair, and growth. For a true working knowledge of why you eat what you eat, it helps to understand them as more than just names on a food information table, but in relation to their origin, form, and use in your body.

Protein

Protein is made up of chains of amino acids, the building blocks of living cells, and can be found in animal sources, but also in beans, nuts, dairy products, and even grains and vegetables. The primary use for protein is to reconstruct and build tissues in your body, but when carbohydrates run low or when you have fasted for even a modest amount of time, protein is also broken down by your body for fuel (the energy found in their molecular bonds).

Doing so comes at a great cost metabolically, however. Burning protein for fuel, as many low-carb devotees do, is kind of like burning the furniture to heat the house. It works, but there are easier fuels to use, and you just lost a nice sofa.

We get more than enough protein in the American diet, which is why protein loading and the focus on protein in so many "performance foods" today may often present marketing-driven overkill. The protein powders used by bodybuilders often contain whey, a protein that is extracted from milk during the production process. This fact makes protein powders not nearly as complex as their multisyllabic names would imply, but it also makes it hard to justify the expense of their production, much less the industrial-size tubs they often come packaged in. There are reasons to use protein for non-nutritive purposes related to sports nutrition, however, and these have little to do with getting a neck that can break bricks. These will be discussed later in the chapter.

Carbohydrates

Carbohydrates—carbon and hydrogen hexagons when put under the microscope—show up in plant, fruit, and vegetable matter. Unlike fat and protein, we can't put carbohydrates to work as repair material for our tissues, as the body has virtually no parts made of carbohydrates. Rather, carbohydrates are only stripped for parts during metabolism—they are loot your body ransacks for the high-energy bonds used to keep those carbon and hydrogen atoms connected, energy which it then uses to *reconnect* the ATP molecules necessary for powering muscular contractions. In addition to voluntary and involuntary muscle movements and heat, your body also needs carbohydrates to fuel the electrical activity of the brain. Carbohydrates are stored in the blood in the form of glucose, which keeps the brain working. They are stored in the muscles in the form of glycogen, to fuel movement.

The carbohydrates you consume in excess of the small amount needed to keep your brain working for four hours, are stored in the liver and in little garages throughout your muscles. These holding places can hold only so many carbohydrates, and once those are full and your blood sugar is at its maximum, your body will take the rest of any carbohydrates you eat and convert them into the second category of food found in nature, the lipid acids known as fats.

Dietary Fats

You can create body fat from your dietary carbs, but somehow we have historically directed most of our nutritional attention toward the subject of whether or not we should be eating fat. As a nutritional focus, the low-fat perspective is overemphasized in this regard, because once it gets in your tissues, fat is fat, and carbohydrate-derived fats are the same as fat-derived fat. Unlike carbohydrates, dietary fats are found in both animal and plant matter, and are needed by the body for cell repair (they form the outer barrier to the cell), organ insulation, and storage as fuel.

Fats are energy dense—they generate more heat per unit of measure than other sources of energy. This characteristic makes them ideal for fueling aerobic activity, which requires a long, sustained burn

to cover the dozens of biochemical steps necessary to reconnect ATP through oxygen-aided metabolism. More pressing to our diet, however, is the fact of our inborn urge regarding energy density. We have evolved to crave such "energy-dense" foods—or at least find them pleasing to the palette—because those who consume them are better equipped to survive famine. This primal preference for energy-dense foods works for us in a condition of scarcity, but has gotten us into XXXL sweatpants in two shakes of a stick, evolution-wise, in a food environment flush with cheap and tasty energy-dense foods. One less-heralded benefit of dietary fat is that it promotes satiety. It is easier to feel full when you have consumed some fat, and that makes you stop eating.

The Misunderstood World of Fat

Fat has long been seen as the bad guy in nutrition, but it turns out that while all fats are calorically dense, not all fats are bad for you. Fats are classified according to their hydrogen content, and this greatly influences how the body is affected by them. So-called "monounsaturated" fats (derived from sources like nuts, olive oil, canola oil, and avocados) are good for you. Though they do have the same caloric liability of being as energy dense as every other form of fat, olive and nut oils do not raise your bad cholesterol, and they actually lower your good cholesterol. Other fats however, tend to raise your bad cholesterol: polyunsaturated fats (derived from vegetable oils) do so, albeit to a lesser degree than saturated fats (derived from animal fat and coconut oil). "Partially hydrogenated" or *trans*-fats (derived from certain plant oils and found in many commercially prepared crackers, cookies, chips, cereals, popcorn, breads, peanut butter, and margarines) were designed to stay firm at room temperature and to go easier on your bad cholesterol, yet they are some of the worst fats for your health. Finally, your body actually needs certain types of fat—the so-called omega-3 fatty acids found in salmon, trout, fish oils, and flaxseed. They help to keep your brain healthy and reduce your risk of heart disease.

With these many nuanced, fat-separating distinctions in mind, it's little surprise that the connection between eating fat and storing fat has turned out not to be as simple as many once believed. During the 1970s and 1980s American food companies churned out a broad range of low-fat foods, but to make up for the fats they extracted, these foods often added more sugar, which, like fat, is also energy dense. In those cases where they do not add sugar but make a fat-tasting product, the artificial fillers often fail to perform at promoting satiety, another liability of skipping the real thing. As a result, the low-fat food era saw fat content of most treats drop but the caloric content change little, and Americans became fatter than ever.

For years it was thought that eating fat put you at greater risk of storing fat, but this may have turned out to be a mistaken assumption of fuel storage. The body can turn excess lima bean- and whole-grain calories into fat just as easily as it can butter calories. It's just really hard to eat excess calories in bulky, fiber-stuffed foods like whole grains and lima beans. It's almost impossible. The low-fat diets saw their influence wane with the arrival 10 years ago of the low-carb era, a host of diets that pointed the finger at carbohydrates as the real bad guy in nutrition. Blaming all carbs however, is also a grave oversimplification, one just now being cleared up with diets that promote the selective eating of "good" carbohydrates. One reason so many are now willing to implicate carbohydrates in weight problems has to do with a recent discovery about them: When we grind them too small, they wreak metabolic havoc over time.

Weight Management Rules

When dealing with weight-management issues, there are three basic rules of eating you should follow: Choose slow-burning carbs, choose food with low-caloric density, and eat small meals often.

Rule # 1: Choose Slow-Burning Carbs

Food companies have milled grains to ever smaller (hence smoother and "tastier") particulate size over the years, and the result has been carbohydrates that act more like energy-dense fats. A soft piece of bread may taste sweet on the palate, but its finely milled carbohydrates are often broken down so quickly in the gut that they flood the veins with glucose, unleashing a doubly troubling chain reaction that causes you first to underutilize what you do eat, and second, to eat again sooner than you would otherwise.

The body is one big chain of biochemical transactions, and the transaction created by the arrival of a sudden rush of blood sugar from a fast-burning carbohydrate is a crisis. There is an ensuing release of the hormone insulin, which turns the glucose into fat for storage, mutes response to insulin over time and causes your blood supply to become prematurely depleted of glucose. In this circumstance—the "crash" that happens 20 minutes after eating fast-burning sugars—you have enough calories to function but your body thinks otherwise. As a result, you get hungry earlier than you should, thereby instilling the consumption of ever more calories. The reality of fast-burning carbohydrates may be a little more nuanced—excess carbohydrates often just linger for future fuel, slowing your burning of fuel—but as Chris Carmichael writes in *Food for Fitness* "the end result is the same." More fat is stored.

Fortunately, a scale has been devised to help with the identification of fast-burning carbohydrates, and it is known as the glycemic index. The glycemic index rates foods on a scale of 1–100, with the foods that are converted to sugar the fastest scoring the highest, and those that digest slower, scoring lower. Foods that score high on the glycemic index include most white and sticky foods with a high starch content, such as large baked potatoes, white bread, white rice, and soft pasta. The glycemic index is filled with its own idiosyncrasies: "junk" foods with added sugar like candy and sweetened cereal often score lower than "natural" foods like potatoes, simply because table sugar in junk foods retains water in the stomach, and this water slows digestion. Moreover, it can be hard to extrapolate from individual glycemic values how an entire meal will digest in combination; your fat-laden pudding could slow down the glycemic effect of your fast-burning dinner roll. But it is safe to say the attention paid to the effects of fast-burning carbohydrates on your satiety and ener-gy level is critical in managing caloric consumption.

Consider the glycemic index when shopping for your starches, *not* your fats, treats, proteins, or fruits and vegetables. (The glycemic ratings on some vegetables such as carrots are high, but it is an anomaly of testing; you would have to eat an extraordinary amount to spike your blood sugar.) Even many of the "bad" foods do not need to be prohibited, merely eaten in moderation and with care given to their preparation. In many cases this could mean simply substituting parboiled rice for white rice (parboiling changes the nature of the starch), red potatoes for large russets, cooking pasta more firmly than softly, and eating whole-grain breads and cereals instead of soft white or brown breads and highly processed cereals.

Rule #2: Choose Foods with Low Caloric Density

The real currency of nutritional knowledge is calories, of course, or the amount of heat generated by burning a gram of a given food source. You need calories in order to function, lest your body raid your fat and muscle tissue, but the amount your body needs before storing the rest is anyone's guess. The typical range often given is 1500–2000 calories daily, but a large male can require 3000 or more calories a day without storing fat or raiding stores, and athletes can require even more.

Caloric intake in America has been rising steadily for decades, as portion sizes, calorically dense options that do not make you satisfied until you have eaten too many, and other preparation factors all overload the body with more energy than it can use.

According to Barry Popkin, a professor of nutritional anthropology at the University of North Carolina–Chapel Hill, the primary change in the American diet has been a shift from eating 90 percent of our calories at home to eating 45–50 percent of our calories at home. Eating out, of course, is to place yourself in the hands of an industry that has literally used the term "wow factor" to describe the way they can, for a fraction of the cost, double a portion size and freak you out so much you want to come back again and again. Studies show that people will tend to eat what's on their plate, no matter the size, and in the process of years of being wowed by the food industry, our understanding of what constitutes a portion has changed. Check out the desserts they are selling at the dinner house chains sometime. Or the muffins at diners. These things are as big as your head, good eatin' too. At least until the chair gives out and you have to give the manager your credit card.

Much of the caloric overload in America today has to do with the way we artificially delay our natural shutoff mechanism, through the consumption of calorically dense foods. It used to be fairly difficult to obtain very many grams of energy-dense foods—to squeeze juice and to dry fruits, extract sugars, reduce syrups, separate cream from milk, and extract oil from plants. As a result, in days past our diet warranted less concern over excessive consumption of energy-dense foods. Today however, tightly compacted calories are not only more readily available, they are the foods easiest to sell and often cheapest to produce.

This may be the way of Big Food in America today, but the human appetite evolved in response to foods in their natural form. Our metabolism was developed in the presence of unprocessed whole foods—whole grains, fruits, and vegetables. The benefits of eating whole foods isn't due to vitamins. Hardly anyone has a vitamin deficiency in the western world today. You need whole foods, rather, for their colors, which carry with them different active properties that help keep your body working at its peak. But primarily you need whole foods for two rather ordinary ingredients, the two things that best promote a feeling of satiety—water and fiber.

Research shows that we push away from the table not when we reach a certain number of calories, but when our stomach is full. This happens much sooner after eating whole grain foods, fresh fruits and vegetables, soups, and other prepared foods composed with the fiber and water. The authorities tell you to get a certain number of servings of fruits and vegetables, but they might as well just say that every meal should have whole foods in it and spare you all the dreary work of portion counting.

Conversely, while whole foods have in common a high percentage of fiber and water, the vast majority of what is offered for sale from the packaged food industry offers you exactly the opposite. Because they are harder to process, store, and ship, the one thing most prepared foods and juices share is a near banishment of these two ingredients. You can buy nearly anything you want in the center aisles of a typical American grocery store except foods filled with water and fiber. Because of these conditions, the more processed food you eat, the more calories you will need to eat

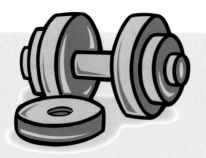

TO CONTROL CALORIC CREEP, BEWARE SWEETENED BEVERAGES

O f all processed foods, one food in particular gets us in caloric trouble. The rise of sweetened beverage and juice consumption adds new calories to our diet, calories which, unlike many other convenience foods, tend to not be subtracted from our caloric total at the next meal time. If you consume 120 calories in a glass of milk, for example, your body tends to need that many fewer calories when you eat a meal. If you consume 120 calories in a bottled sweet drink, however, the body wants to eat the same amount of calories it would have needed if you had never popped the top in the first place. The high-fructose corn syrup used in most commercially prepared beverages is the sweetener least likely to leave us feeling satisfied. But it pales in comparison to the larger effect of adding calories from beverages, which have little net effect on satisfying hunger.

before feeling full, and you will likely get fatter.

Rule # 3: Eat Small Meals Often

Switching over to starches with a lower glycemic index value, and eating more low-caloric-density whole foods are two low-maintenance ways to control what you eat for the better. Without any complicated formulas to remember or meta-nutrient balances to keep track of, both can be accomplished simply by shifting your consumption to foods that exist in as unprocessed a form as possible. This can be assisted by some targeted changes in your daily order. Chances are to eat more whole foods you need to try new foods on a regular basis; you need to shop for fresh foods two to three times a week—(preferably at those smaller specialty-food stores that make frequent shopping easier to pull off); you need to plan ahead so you have fresh foods at the ready around the kitchen; and you need to budget the time to cook. There are certain prepared foods that can help you eat fresh foods as well—frozen cut vegetables and berries are great to have on hand.

But there is one last piece to the weight-management puzzle, and it too requires little in the way of formula memorization or calorie counting. It is the importance of not restricting. So much focus has been placed on eating less, when the real concern is to eat less of energy-dense foods. To the contrary, simply eating less can be a real prescription for weight gain. Quite simply, the body needs foods every three to four hours, and to wait longer, as our three squares a day culture encourages, has a number of consequences: it invites the temporary raiding of protein stores instead of fat; it slows down your ability to burn fat, and it leaves you to eat in a satiety-compromised state that will encourage eating more total calories than you would have eaten had you simply had a light snack.

The solution: Instead of the typical 600-, 800-, 1,000-calorie meal plan for breakfast, or worse yet, a skipped breakfast, 600-calorie lunch, 2,000-calorie dinner, and 500 calories to get you through *Law & Order*, try to eat more smaller meals throughout the day. Divide your breakfast in half and eat it at 7:00 and 10:00. Do the same with your lunch at noon and 3:00. Eat dinner, though slightly less than normal and then have a snack before bed. This works out to roughly a 300, 300, 550, 250, 700, 300-calorie plan.

SPORTS NUTRITION

With so much to learn about how to stay out of weight trouble, it seems like a luxury to get to the point in the conversation where you talk about how to make food work in a training plan. If you are at this point, congratulations, you are miles ahead of most of us. The primary goals of sport nutrition come down to five things:

- How to make sure you have the most possible energy at the start of a workout or race

- How to make sure you don't suffer any stomach cramping during a workout or race

- How to make sure you take in enough energy during a workout or race to replenish that which was lost

- How to hydrate so that you will neither become dehydrated, flushed of salts, nor overhydrated

- How to use nutrition to enable you to work out again sooner once you are done

That said, there is more than meets the eye when it comes to sports nutrition. There are a host of products competing for your dollars and a lot of confusing research to account for, starting with the way many of the rules about food get reversed once you lace up your shoes and start to sweat.

The Paradox of Fast-Burning Carbs

Remember how we said not to eat fast-burning carbs? Well, forget all that. . . . The sports nutrition business has been booming over the last several years, churning out a variety of gels, bars, drinks, and powders to help get you through your workout. If you look at the ingredient list of most of these products, knowing what we know about insulin-spiking, fast-burning carbohydrates, you would think these sweetener-laden products are some of the worst things you could consume before a workout. If they make you crash and get hungry too soon just while sitting at your desk, imagine the havoc they would wreak on your run!

But it turns out that the insulin spike and blood-sugar crash that accompanies the ingestion of fast-burning carbohydrates while at rest, does *not* occur when the body is working at a sustained, vigorous activity level. Basically, during extended work efforts your body is working hard enough that the sugar is utilized as it enters your bloodstream, and does not generally overload your system to the point where an insulin overload is delivered from your pancreas. To the contrary, one of the *best* things you can do for your body is to offer it fast-burning carbohydrates while working out for a period of an hour or longer. It may be great to give your body its carbohydrates in the form of slow-to-digest fresh produce while at rest, but place these in a stomach that is deprived of blood flow (blood is redirected to your legs when training) and it would only invite abdominal cramping.

Indeed, most "energy" products, be they bars, gels, powders, or drinks are merely potable preparations of high-glycemic carbohydrates. For this reason, a can of Coke has many of the same benefits to offer an athlete as a bottle of a sports drink; a tablespoon of honey or pudding shares many of the same benefits of a sports gel, and a sandwich generally acts the same in your body as many energy bars. Your body will benefit from gels or high-glycemic beverages for workouts longer than an hour in duration. You can take them as early as a half hour into the workout.

Another Paradox—
Caffeine Helps Endurance

Just as high-glycemic carbohydrates do one thing while at rest and another while exercising vigorously, research now suggests that caffeine is handled by your body with a similar versatility depending upon whether you are working out or not. Because it acts as a diuretic—it causes you to pee—nutritionists have long warned against ingesting caffeine during a workout. On paper this makes sense, as diuretics make you dehydrated while at rest and avoiding dehydration is the primary objective of sports nutrition. But some research now suggests that caffeine not only does *not* cause dehydration when working at a sustained elevated pace, it may actually promote better endurance performance. It does make sense, anecdotally at least. Chances are drinking a Diet Coke before a stint at the desk has caused you to need to pee, while doing so before a hard run does not. The fluid shifts at work in your body change the effect of caffeine on your water-retention systems. Researchers are not sure exactly why caffeine actually helps endurance performance, but some think it is possible the drug acts to buffer either the perception of pain or the actual feeling of pain, giving you the psychological boost to go a little longer.

How to Load

Sports nutrition is commonly organized around either those foods that aid in sustaining endurance efforts or those that promote strength training. For those who are about to run, the common wisdom has changed little; you do not want to run hungry, and you do not want to run full. Eating an hour before a run is the easiest solution, ideally slow-burning carbohydrates such as oatmeal or whole-grain breads. Just immediately prior to a run you can ingest some quick-burning carbohydrates for a boost, though for those watching their weight this is really necessary only for those about to run for an extensive length of time. Last but not least there is the question of how to ensure that your glycogen stores are at their peak just prior to running in an all-out endurance effort such as an organized race. To do this, athletes have commonly showed up for night-before spaghetti dinners, but the backstory is that the best effect of carbohydrate loading is achieved when you taper your consumption of carbohydrates at the start of the week prior to a race to deplete your stores, then increase them to three quarters of your calories in the two days prior. Clearly, none of this falls in line with the low-carbohydrate trend that has swept the country over the last several years, nor should it. Athletes burn carbohydrates, and require more than most of us. Cutting back on them just doesn't make a lot of sense for training.

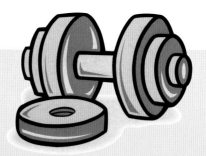

RESTRICTING

In the pursuit of thinness, many people try to use willpower to deny themselves food, either by skipping meals or eating very little. What happens to these restrictors, unfortunately, is that once the body goes for too long without food, it responds by temporarily slowing down its metabolism. Restricting ultimately causes a short-term slowdown in the rate at which your body burns energy at rest—the resting metabolic rate—(RMR). The body can become so confused due to restriction that girls with eating disorders have been known to stop menstruating—a sign the body is starving—while remaining overweight according to standard weight tables. As a population that restricts, the study of anorexics can tell us much about ordinary restriction. Studies have shown that those who exercise on top of this type of restriction have even slower metabolisms.

Restriction also causes your body to burn protein disproportionately, which is hardly the goal of someone trying to trim that fat off their thighs. Georgia State University researcher Dan Benardot monitored elite gymnasts and distance runners to see how often they ate each day. His team was the first to look at variations in energy deficits through the course of a day, and found that the hungrier the athletes got before eating, the higher their body fat percentage. You will actually burn muscle when you are hungry, and your body will conserve its fat, as if in a famine. Indeed, anorexics who die of the disease have some of the highest body fat percentages of anyone, simply because they have lost so much muscle. In contrast, frequent eating is linked with lower body fat percentage, fewer stress hormones, and less insulin response, says Benardot. Lastly, when someone who has restricted does finally eat, in the short term there are other consequences: The body has turned off the "full" meter, causing you to eat far more total calories than you would have in two smaller meals combined. You simply can't mess around with this powerful internal energy shutoff mechanism. Research shows again and again that the more people diet, the more they weigh.

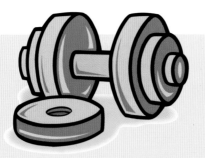

THE RECOVERY WINDOW AND PROTEIN

Researchers have learned there is a window following the conclusion of a workout when your body is more amenable to replenishing its depleted glycogen stores. In the 45 minutes following a workout, some argue, it is easier for glucose to be converted into muscle glycogen. That alone has done much to spur the growth of athletes consuming recovery beverages following a workout, as it is not always easy to get to your fridge when you are concluding a long cycling or paddling session somewhere. Recently however, these same researchers have begun to produce studies suggesting that including a small amount of protein in your recovery foods can act to leverage even more glycogen into your muscles during this recovery window. Specifically, they cite a four-to-one ratio of carbohydrates to protein as one that provides just the amount of protein needed to maximize your glycogen storage. (Protein acts to leverage more carbohydrates into muscle tissue.) Naturally, these same researchers have produced and marketed drinks that meet this profile, but even one of their original designers says that you can wing it with a turkey sandwich if you want to get a four-to-one carbohydrate-to-protein ratio but don't feel like dropping the money for a fancy recovery beverage. While the whey protein found in recovery beverages does become metabolized quicker, the overall effect of homemade, four-to-one carbohydrate to protein food choices is likely to be much the same.

Protein is also necessary for athletes, simply because muscles are torn down in the training process and need to be rebuilt through rest and nutrition. But aside from those who are trying to build muscle mass, there is little need to go to great lengths to eat more protein than the rest of us. It's in your meat, cheese, nuts, and beans, and in this country, we tend to eat portion sizes of all these proteins far in excess of the levels required.

How to Sustain

During an extensive workout, it's likely you will feel run-down, sluggish, or experience your heart rate climbing while your effort level stays the same. This could be an effect of your level of training, but it also could be the result of your blood sugar or hydration levels dropping. The thing is, your body is not going to tell you, and you owe it to yourself to make sure that isn't the explanation, at least if you are about to quit before you really need to. One way to be sure that your workout isn't suffering from nutrition or dehydration is to be proactive, making a conscious effort to plan for hydration.

To stay on top of your hydration, be sure to drink 8 or so ounces of water 15 minutes before you begin working out, and to have a sip of water every fifteen minutes. (In the high heat elite runners have been known to drink sports drinks for the entire duration.) If you are training for more than an hour, chances are you will need to get some carbohydrates with your hydration as well, and if you are sweating heavily due to heat or your body temperature, after a lengthy period of exertion simply drinking water is counterproductive. The more you sweat, the more your body loses the electrolytes necessary to keep water in your cells. Once these begin to drop, the scales tip at a molecular level within your body's tissues and in a vicious cycle—increasing your water consumption actually starts pulling more water from your cells. This is why sports drinks contain sodium and potassium.

One last factor to consider, and one that has only recently gained attention is the danger of overhydrating while endurance training, a condition known as hyponatremia. Thanks to the crush of interest in preventing dehydration, organized races offer drink tables at frequent intervals and racers are encouraged to drink up. Many runners can actually overdo it with the hydration, however, which can cause its own set of problems. Finding a balance between dehydration and overhydration is individual, but it pays to keep in mind that with water or fluids there is such a thing as too much of a good thing.

How to Recover

The last step of the sports-nutrition process is to replenish your glycogen stores following the completion of a long effort. When you work out for a long period of time you strip your muscles of their stores of glycogen. For a long time it was simply thought that all that mattered to replace missing glycogen was to ingest fast-burning carbohydrates at the completion of a training effort. Recently, however, researchers have begun to argue that there are better ways to do this more effectively. Replenishing your glycogen stores optimally is primarily a question for die-hard training devotees, as your body will replenish most of what you have lost through the normal course of meals within a 24-hour period. But for those who may wish to schedule more than one workout in a day, and the growing numbers of triathletes in our ranks makes that scenario more likely, there is a specific window for replenishment, and a specific ratio believed to improve replenishment (see sidebar).

Like training in general, a sound nutrition plan will ultimately have to work within the rhythms and goals of your life. Indeed, one of the biggest obstacles to most nutrition plans is the way they often attempt to wedge all parties into the sort of endless calorie- and gram- and serving-counting that only a nutritionist could love. But with the larger principles of how to eat in general, and during training in particular, there's no reason people can't use the best of what we know about food to confidently undertake smart, realistic, food choices and attitudes every day of their lives.

chapter 11
REAL LIFE IS COMPLICATED

THE OFFICIAL RECOMMENDATION OF THE AMOUNT OF EXERCISE necessary for Americans to lose weight or stay healthy has risen from 30 to 60 to 90 MINUTES A DAY. In the same breath, HEALTH OFFICIALS ANNOUNCED that Americans

should eat 13 servings of fruits and vegetables a day, another suggestion greeted with spit-takes at kitchen tables across America. There isn't even enough produce in the nation's food supply to cover the *old* recommendation.

There is a growing disconnect between the things we do and the things we are supposed to do. While each of these arguments for raising the bar on how much we should exercise makes sense, simply telling us to do more without telling us how to make that happen is a recipe for discouragement. And no matter what you think about the touchy-feely business of not wanting to make other people discouraged, it is hardly conducive to getting more activity out of people.

In this regard, one of the most important things you can do to improve your chances of getting in shape—even more important than going to the gym—is to direct your attention toward the human factors of training. You can't really think

about training without thinking about the realities of how your life will interrupt all your good intentions (repeatedly and with great creativity and innovation) over and over throughout your life. You will get injured, you will get sick, you will fall off

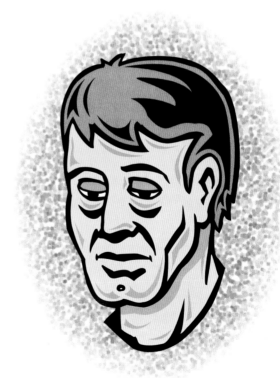

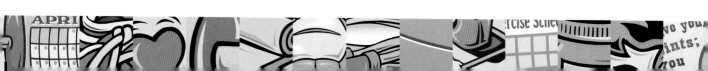

the wagon, you will go on business trips, vacations, change jobs, get relocated, get lazy, enter new relationships, and take on new responsibilities, and all of these passages will have an effect on your success at staying active for life. To be resilient in the face of this certainty, more than anything else, will mean making a habit out of managing your life for success.

There are more than a few really talented people out there to tell you about the head game of motivation, the mental obstacles to activity that you put in place for yourself and how to overcome them. Indeed, a good attitude or outlook will do more to increase your chances of success than almost anything. But habits of thought and behavior can affect your outlook. Good habits can make your future look bright just as readily as bad habits can darken the skies. For example, you can try to fight depression through a number of medical or introspective interventions, but one simple behavioral habit has been shown to reduce depression: writing down three things that went well at the end of each day and why. The way in which we think about our goals, can also be thought of as a habit.

CLEARING YOUR MENTAL ENVIRONMENT

Just as you take the time to organize the environment on your desk to pay bills on time, you can better organize the environment in your head. Your thoughts are far less mystical than you might think, say a growing school of behavioral psychologists who spend their time getting people to look at their automatic thoughts—habits of thinking that can be made to set you up for a better chance of success.

Releasing Your Reckless Rigidity

This book has tried to couch its advice in language that conveys a sense of flexibility about what you need to do to become more fit, and not simply because the author has a chip on his shoulder about rigid protocols, the engineering-like mental orientation common in outdoors sports, and pretty much anyone in a position of authority. It's because in many ways, having the discipline to be flexible is more harmonious with the transformation toward integrating fitness into your life.

Flexibility is key to the very nature of how we approach change in activity level. Research shows that we are always in one of five basic fitness status categories:

- Precontemplation, where we aren't in training and don't think we need to be

- Contemplation, where we think we need to do more but have not

- Preparation, where we train, but only intermittently

- Action, where we train regularly but have only done so for six months

- Maintenance, where we exercise regularly and have done so for more than six months

Research shows that we routinely move from one category to another and back and forward again. We cycle in and out of the activity consistency we think we should always possess, but we are always in one of those five categories. While there is a wonderful consistency to our inconsistency, if you look at your training through an all-or-nothing, highly rigid perspective you may use any of these transitions as a reason to quit. So a rigid perspective is part of your mental environment that needs to be altered to allow success: You may not be able to become a little pregnant, but you *can* be a little invested in a training plan, and indeed, you have to be in order to get started.

A rigid thinking style is surely a central factor to overcome when trying to ensure a more sustainable approach to training, but there are a host of small ways to change this part of your outlook:

- Accept the possibility that your time commitment may rise and fall and rise again through the months and years, but that the commitment itself will not change.

- Accept the possibility that you may need to try different sports to keep your interest level up.

- Accept the possibility that you can work in short durations.

- Accept the fact that you can train in shorter blocks of time, in a variety of surroundings, and under a variety of conditions in your home and work life.

Releasing the "Shoulds" and "Musts"

It helps to know why you are training of course, and you do that by setting goals that are both specific and personally meaningful. A sustainable approach is one that is specific—say, training three to four times per week for six weeks—without being so specific that it loses a personal connection to your life—like a goal of simply losing 10 pounds. This also means developing goals that are based on more than vague assertions that you *must* or *should* do anything. Albert Ellis, the great behavioral psychologist and creator of rational emotive therapy describes *should* and *must* as two words that do little more than make people feel bad about themselves and less likely to accomplish their goals. He calls "must," "musterbation." He says that saying "should here, and should there, and pretty soon there's should all over the place." He's got a colorful way of describing human folly. But his point is powerful—that simply releasing yourself of the notion that anyone *must* or *should* do anything frees up an enormous amount of wasted psychological energy. At the very least, the sooner you stop saying the words in relation to others, the better you will feel about the state of affairs in your life. More to the point, every time the words *should* or *must* enter your mind in relation to yourself, try replacing them with *want*. If you are telling yourself you should do something that you can't say you want to do, you quickly realize you need a better reason. If you can say you *want* to do something like train, replacing thoughts of obligation with thoughts of desire turns an action-stifling perspective into one that makes taking action more likely.

Chasing a State of Mind

Hopefully, replacing *should* with *want* will help open your mind up to your real sources of motivation. Often people will take up a training plan thinking their goal is to drop 20 pounds. But try to show up at a gym day after day with some number on a scale as your only goal. Chances are that goal does not motivate you nearly as much as what the experience of actually living fitter would do for you. *Living* fitter—since you live it, day after simple day, rather than achieve it—would get you not to care so much about the whole big issue of 20 pounds this way or that. Living fitter would get your mind on better things, like the water, the woods, the rock, and the sand—or better yet, other people, places, lives, and questions far more interesting than those of your small dance with exercise. Try simply to embrace work, sweat, a little soreness, and the privilege of being able to move, quickly, lastingly, and powerfully. Get greedy about getting some of that good stuff, and you have a goal that doesn't disappear when you start buying a different size of pants.

The Specificity of Progress

Lest a larger journey toward living fitter seem a tad vague, there is no harm in coming up with goals based on very specific experiences. Contrary to popular belief, there is no harm in striving to accomplish something very ambitious physically. As triathlete and motivator Eric Harr says, thinking big is sometimes just the thing to banish your self-imposed limitations, and you can always scale back your goals at a later time. Maybe your specific goal is showing up to train three days a week for four months. Maybe your specific goal is increasing the speed at which you can run for a half hour by 30 seconds per mile. Maybe your specific goal is getting to the point where you can push, pull, squat, lunge, extend, and rotate your body weight in 3 sets of 20. In other words, there is a lot of mental downtime on a path toward consistency, and if you are at all prone to losing focus, having specific benchmarks at the start are far better enticements than a subjective goal such as getting yourself a box of rocks in your abs. Talk about goalposts that are likely to move further away the closer you get . . .

A PHYSICAL ENVIRONMENT FOR SUCCESS

Changing the framework for how you set goals and evaluate your progress will do much to improve the likelihood of sustainable activity in your life. Changing your physical environment is another great way to help your chances of living actively. Stated as simply as possible, you want to make training as easy as possible, in every environment, according to every turn of your schedule. We are products of our surroundings far more than we realize, and it is clear that simply improving your logistical ease of staying active will improve your likelihood of staying active. There is no shortage of ways to clear a path for activity consistency.

Time

Have some breakfast first, but try to train early if at all possible. There are innumerable obligations that can arise as the day goes along, but the very start of the day is the time that is least likely to be encroached upon by other responsibilities. The corollary to training at 7:00 or earlier of course, is the need to be realistic about getting enough sleep. The two go together. You probably can't work with the dawn and still watch the late news, much less *Nightline,*

Dave, Jay, or yikes, Conan. If going to bed early feels strange, stay up as late as usual and show up at the gym for a couple of days before 7:00 on less sleep. You will get so exhausted that falling asleep earlier in the evening will take care of itself. That said, there are those who have to work late, have to work early, or simply can't stand the idea of training before their brain has been turned on for a few hours. Noon, after work, or early evening are all the same to your body. You can even stagger your workouts at different points in the day throughout the week. What matters is that you go.

Consistency

Get a partner if at all possible. Having someone you're accountable to on days when you would rather do other things is one of the few factors shown to increase exercise participation. More important, it is even more beneficial if your partner is someone who shares compatible goals, and even challenges you. If your partner is at a more or less advanced stage of training than are you, run your own pace and catch up to, or wait for him or her at the end. Sharing the ride there and home is an incentive all its own. Run your own pace and don't compare yourselves. All work is relative. Slow-moving intensity is the same as fast-moving intensity, it's just a few months or years behind on the training arc.

Gear

Whenever possible, get good gear. If you want to spend time every day in a training activity, you owe it to yourself to do whatever you can to make the experience more enjoyable. Good shoes, training clothes, and workout gear can lift the quality of

your experience measurably, by helping your body breathe, stay warm, stay cool, cushioned, and protected. If you are lifting, get gloves. If you are running, have your stride checked out to see if you need a stabilizing shoe or a cushioning shoe. If you live in rainy or snowy weather, get the gear necessary to allow you to train in the entire range of conditions for where you live, be it cold, snow, heat, rain, or wind. Have enough gear to have some in the wash and some in the bag. Keep your gear separate, and in an easy place to get at both in the dark and in a hurry. Get a bag and keep it in your car, in case you need to sneak in a workout on the fly. Keep a fridge full of sport drinks in the garage. Keep a set of dumbbells, a jump rope, yoga mat, rubber medicine ball, and a fitness bar in a spare room at home as well, for the days when you can't get out of the house. Splurge on an MP3 player and give yourself some music to make the time go faster. Allow yourself a new CD for every month you stick to your workout. Try not to do all of this on credit. Your spouse or banker will get upset with you and the stress will interfere with your ability to enjoy your runs!

Location

If you are going to use a club, find a club near your work, and don't be afraid to find a second, cheaper club to use for those times when you are burned out on the first one. Learn the mileage and location of the local paved pathways, wooded trails, and country roads. Scout out new places to ride, run, or ski on weekends, using your car odometer to mark out parking places, starting and stopping points, and the length of the ride from home. Avoid running routes that are home to lots of traffic, noise, and busy intersections that are just going to make you stressed out. Pick out visually enticing places to train whenever possible. On weekends, get up early and drive to scenic training destinations that are even more enticing.

Scheduling

If you have no time to train, and hence you never train, something has to go. Start with TV, if you haven't already. Chances are you only watch TV at night, but if you watch it in the morning, there you go—use that time and leave the cartoons for the demographic for whom they were intended. Simply by not turning it on, you will feel antsy from the quiet. Listen to that antsyness, and use it to get moving into your goal. If you watch TV late into the night, that may seem like free time, but think of it as time taken away from your training time in the morning. If you use TV to wind down before bed, try turning down your lights after dinner, stopping thinking about work, taking a warm bath, and reading. You will be snoozing before you know it, and probably save on your outlays for imported beer as well.

Is your family time or relationship time running low? Make going to the club a his and her or family activity. Are you running lots of errands during your weekday after work? Consolidate your extracurricular activities on the weekends, or better yet, pare them down. Quit your clubs, quit overscheduling your child, buy less stuff (except good gear!), lower your expectations about the state of your house, car, or wardrobe. If you have all that and you have no active life, those things will be cold comfort anyway. Are you eating too much at lunch? Leave the job a half hour earlier, eat something light, and train the rest of the time. You will have more energy in the late afternoon and your extra productivity will make up for the extra half hour you took off. Or at least that's what you can tell your boss.

It's easy to get caught up in the latest idea of what exercises to do, how often to do them, how many times and when precisely you should grunt and groan, but the technical information related to training is mostly oversold. Managing your thoughts and your life to permit an active life is far more critical. Take the time to create a mental and physical environment for success at staying active and you just may get a chance to test out those dumbbells gathering dust in your garage.

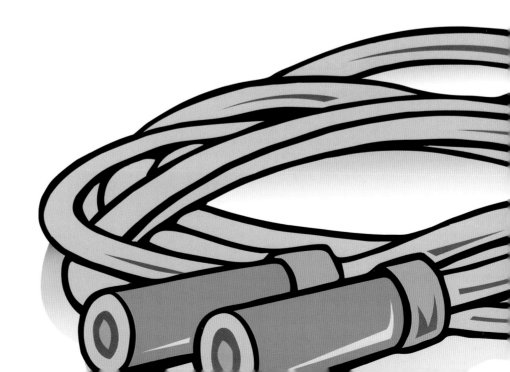

chapter 12

50 RULES OF TRAINING

THE TRUTH IS, DESIGNING TRAINING PLANS IS A SCIENCE,

but an IMPROVISATIONAL one based on a handful of principles.

Here's a compilation of these principles, THE BEST OF THE

GOLDEN AGE OF EXERCISE SCIENCE.

Learn them and you can improvise your own smart, effective, individual, and purposeful workouts.

THE RULES

1. Create a goal that's not a number (160 pounds), or a look (rock-solid abs), but a state of mind or an achievement. The number and the look will follow.

2. Periodize. Vary your workouts, organize their objectives over blocks of weeks and months, work in discrete phases of intensity, and reduce your intensity downward 1 level for every 3 levels you step upward. Regular patterns of scaling back and then exploding forward is necessary to keep the body from becoming desensitized to training.

3. Strength grows during recovery. Schedule recovery time within each workout week and month, or schedule burnout.

4. It's all good. Ten minutes 3 times a day equals 30 minutes at once.

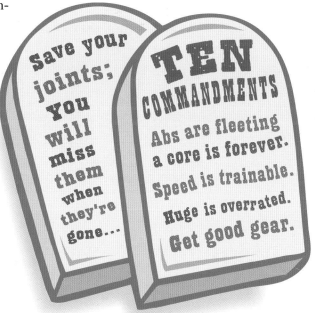

Save your joints; you will miss them when they're gone...

TEN COMMANDMENTS

Abs are fleeting a core is forever.

Speed is trainable.

Huge is overrated.

Get good gear.

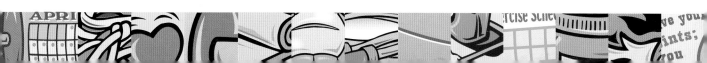

5. You want to know what's aggressive? Aggressive is warming up first, cooling down afterward.

6. To build endurance, count minutes, not miles. And go easy—at just over half of your ability—for a long time, 4–5 days a week, for at least one season.

7. When you feel ready, go for longer. But limit your increases in duration to 10 percent, and every other week.

8. To boost endurance, work with intensity. Mix in short sessions—from 3–10 minutes—at just above and below 75 percent of your ability (or your lactate threshold heart rate). This is a reward for having put in 3 to 4 months of long, slow, distance running.

9. When the short sessions get easy, increase the number of intervals (up to 6) then their length (up to 10 minutes), then start decreasing the rests in between. Try to reduce your breaks from twice the duration of your intervals, to even in duration, to half the duration of your intervals.

10. If you're in the saddle, or pool, try to go longer than if you are running. Non-load-bearing workouts (cycling, swimming) are often twice as long as running workouts.

11. Pressed for time? Try jumping rope.

12. Want to race? Put in the miles. One month beforehand you need to be able to run, swim, or cycle 75 percent as much as you will on race day.

13. You need to be rested to be peaked. To be at your very best, taper down your workload starting at 4 weeks before a competition, and mostly rest the last 2.

14. Everyone has to build strength, even runners, even swimmers, even you.

15. Work the core first.

16. Work the core some more.

17. Train movements (stepping, squatting, pushing, pulling, extending, and rotating), not body parts.

18. Three lifts done with good form is more productive than 30 done sloppy. It'll also help keep you out of the physical therapist's office.

19. If you're new to the lift, your fibers are hurtin'. One set is fine.

20. Iron looks cool, but your body weight is often more than enough (i.e., lunges, pull-ups, squats).

21. When you do go to free weights, use dumbbells as much as possible. They may be small but they're safer, and generally more challenging and functional than barbells.

22. For the world outside of bodybuilding, the down lift is often more important than the up lift. Let it down with control and in a smooth motion.

23. Machines make you strong at machines. Benches make you strong at working from a bench. Real life requires you to be strong while on your feet. Don't stop at machines or benches. Progress to training for ground-based strength.

24. Bending? Bend your knees and pull in your abs.

25. Rotating? Lead with your pelvis, and let your heels turn.

26. Keep your hips above your knees, your thighs to parallel, and your knees behind your toes if you ever want to ski again.

27. Two numbers, 10 and 20. For muscular strength, lift enough weight to wipe you out around 10 reps. For new movements, 20.

28. Stretching is a workout itself, not a wrap-up. Learn the poses of the Sun Salutation. Find a time when you are warm and focused and build your endurance for flexibility.

29. Work slow, be slow: If you need to ever be strong and fast, remember to consider plyometrics, throws, and agility drills.

30. Whenever possible, take it outdoors.

31. Work out in the morning.

32. Have a buddy.

33. Do as little as necessary to get the effect.

34. Have a workout you can do at home.

35. Have a plan with enough variety to keep you interested.

36. Make time to train at the speed you need to do work in life.

37. Train in multiple-joint movements as much as possible. A leg extension, concentration curl, or hamstring curl looks little like how you actually move.

38. Let a muscle rest for 36 hours after resistance training.

39. If possible, strength train 3 times a week (research shows once is generally too little, a fourth visit makes no difference).

40. Practice active stretches. Instead of just propping a muscle into a stretch, pull it into place of its opposing muscle.

41. Cycling? Power monitors make a more efficient use of your training time.

42. Get a heart-rate monitor. It will give you something to think about beside the sound of your feet.

43. Learn your lactate-threshold heart rate. It will make using your monitor more meaningful.

44. Honor the progression. Work from simple to complex, low intensity to high intensity. It is the journey not the destination.

45. If you only have time to work one muscle group it should be your core.

46. Honor the slowing strength in your lower body. It helps deceleration for skiing, down hiking, leaping, and running.

47. Get away from a cardio/strength-training dichotomous view of fitness training. The two systems work together at all times.

48. Practice training that is capable of being maintained for life, by setting some goals.

49. You don't need a brace or belt or super-huge muscles. What you need is a reliable core and stable joints.

50. Start where you are, and you will get to where you want to be.

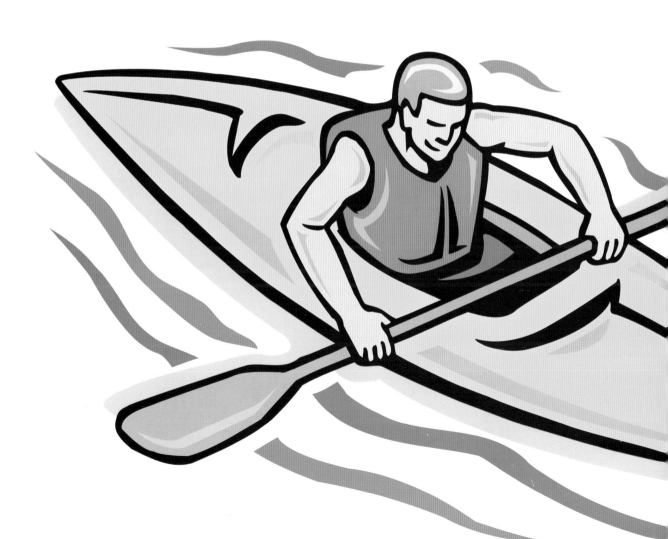

RESOURCES
GUIDE

There's no end to the operations TRYING TO PITCH you products, INFORMATION, AND SERVICES related to fitness. Wandering into this bustling marketplace with only a note from your doctor saying "MUST BECOME FIT" can make a person feel overwhelmed and not a little vulnerable. The following list of fitness-related resources is by no means exhaustive or even necessarily fully endorsed, so USE IT AS A STARTING POINT and use your good judgment. But getting acquainted with the BROAD SPAN OF PLACES TO LEARN about and suit up for training is not only a FIRST STEP towards entering the community of athletes, but part and parcel of DIVING INTO THE ONGOING MYSTERIES OF FITNESS THAT WE TRY TO UNRAVEL DAILY.

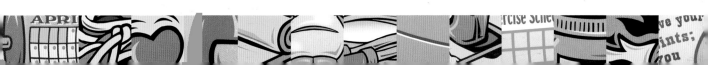

SPORT AND TRAINING ORGANIZATIONS

The American College of Sports Medicine
P.O. Box 1440
Indianapolis, IN 46206-1440
(317) 637-9200
www.acsm.org
The American College of Sports Medicine, a trade organization oversee-ing the medical practice of fitness and sports injury prevention and rehabilita-tion, offers certification, research, and educational materials on training, fit-ness, safety, and injury prevention.

The Cooper Institute
12330 Preston Road
Dallas, TX 75230
(972) 341-3200
www.cooperinst.org
The Cooper Institute, the Texas-based fitness and health research organization is a leading advocate for the benefits of regular aerobic activity and a widely respected authority on exercise and training for health.

The National Academy of Sports Medicine
26632 Agoura Road
Calabasas, CA 91302
(800) 460-6276
www.nasm.org
The National Academy of Sports Medicine is a newer fitness accreditation organization, with an emphasis on strength training emphasizing integrated ("functional") fitness.

The National Strength and Conditioning Association
1885 Bob Johnson Drive
Colorado Springs, CO 80906
(719) 632-6722
www.nsca-lift.org
The National Strength and Conditioning Association is the 30,000-member home for certification and strength-training research and design, a trade association used by coaches and trainers for athletic organizations the world over.

GEAR

Concept2, Inc.
105 Industrial Park Drive
Morrisville, VT 05661
(800) 245-5676
www.concept2.com
Concept2 has expanded the use of the rowing machine, making the act of indoor rowing less isolated and more competitive, by sponsoring large indoor rowing meets, rowing workouts, advice, and other resources.

FaCT Canada Consulting
401 St. Laurent Avenue
Quesnel, BC V2J 5P8
Canada
www.fact-canada.com
This website is home to the primary North American distributorship of Lactate Pro blood lactate analyzer, and also offers power cranks, heart rate mon-itors, and other hardware suitable for those seeking a more precise mastery of their endurance-training protocols.

FreeMotion Fitness
1096 Elkton Drive, Suite 600
Colorado Springs, CO 80907
(877) 363-8449
www.freemotionfitness.com
FreeMotion is a line of machines that put your strength training on your feet and in natural, unrestricted movements via

the use of simple and versatile swivel pulleys and cables. You basically grab a handle and pull a weighted plate in any pathway of your choosing, letting your body's range movement guide the use of the machine, rather than the other way around. Free Motion is not the only manufacturer of cable-based strength training, but they were one of the first to significantly refashion strength machines for greater functionality.

Perform Better
P.O. Box 8090
Cranston, RI 02920-0090
(888) 556-7464
www.performbetter.com
Perform Better is a great one-stop retailing resource for the sorts of tools and coaching materials needed to develop some of the more underappreciated athletic disciplines, including balance, agility, speed, power, and core strength.

Polar Electro, Inc.
1111 Marcus Avenue, Suite M15
Lake Success, NY 11042-1034
(800) 290-6330
www.polarusa.com
Polar brand heart rate monitors are one of the most specialized and innovative providers in the field, with monitor options for beginner and advanced training.

REI
Sumner, WA 98352-0001
(253) 891-2523
www.rei.com
REI outdoor products and gear is a great starting point for everything needed for active training, from heart rate monitors to trail-running shoes.

Sports Resource Group
210 Belmont Road
Hawthorne, NY 10532
(800) 462-2876
www.lactate.com

The Sports Resource Group is the only American distributor of Accutrend Lactate, Lactate Scout, and soon Lactate Plus blood lactate analyzers. These are another option for those hoping to calibrate the presence of lactate in their blood and gauge their improvement in endurance training. The company also offers a rich CD-ROM database of research on the science of how lactic acid affects training.

COACHING AND INSTRUCTION

Beryl Bender Birch
P.O. Box 5009
East Hampton, NY 11937
(631) 324-8409
www.berylbenderbirch.com
The Beryl Bender Birch website offers information about power yoga from this proficient and inspirational New York–based instructor who coined the term.

Carmichael Training Systems
110-B South Sierra Madre
Colorado Springs, CO 80903
(866) 355-0645
www.trainright.com
Carmichael Training Systems offers online coaching, fitness assessment, clinics, gear, and advice under the direction of author and cycling coach Chris Carmichael, coach to Lance Armstrong and leader in the field of individualized, sport-specific aerobic conditioning for cycling, running, multisport, and general fitness.

C.H.E.K. Institute
Sycamore Business Center
2105 Industrial Court
Vista, CA 92081
(800) 552-8789
www.chekinstitute.com
This site is home to the core training seminars, books, and videos developed by Paul Chek, a popular advocate for core development and movement-based training.

Gambetta Sports Training Systems
P.O. Box 50143
Sarasota, FL 34232
(800) 671-4045
www.gambetta.com
Visit this site for seminars, books, and videos related to the movement-based training approach of Vern Gambetta, an original thinker and influential advocate for functional strength and agility development.

Go Swim
102 Sillen Plantation Road
Stevensville, MD 21666
877-467-9461
www.goswim.tv
Go Swim, an online swim coaching resource, offers seminars, articles, and advice about swimming your very best.

Hal Higdon
www.halhigdon.com
Visit this site for the running writer's widely used, race-specific training plans.

House of Speed Inc.
301 Snow Street
Sugar Grove, IL 60554
(877) 827-7333
www.houseofspeed.com

Former NFL receiver Don Beebe's school for speed training offers clinics and other materials for speed development.

The Institute of Human Performance
1950 NW Boca Raton Boulevard
Boca Raton, FL 33432
(561) 620-9556
www.ihpfit.com
The IHP is home to the products and services offered by Juan Carlos Santana, a leading advocate of functional strength development.

Total Immersion Swimming
246 Main Street, Suite 15A
New Paltz, NY 12561
(800) 609-7946
www.totalimmersion.net
Total Immersion, under the direction of Terry Laughlin, has fine-tuned the technique necessary to develop a more "fish-like" stroke, so you will fight the water less and waste less energy.

Ultrafit
11353 East Raintree
Scottsdale, Arizona 85255
(303) 725-4588
www.ultrafit.com
Ultrafit offers online coaching, gear, fitness resources, and articles about training under the direction of author and cycling coach Joe Friel, another widely respected coach for athletes preparing for triathlons, mountain biking, road cycling, and more.

NUTRITION

BMI Calculator
www.bmi-calculator.net/bmr-calculator/
harris-benedict-equation
Look here for the Harris Benedict Equation, a widely recognized calculator to determine daily caloric needs.

Center for Science in the Public Interest
1875 Connecticut Ave. N.W., Suite 300
Washington, D.C. 20009
 (202) 332-9110
www.cspinet.org
The Center for Science in the Public Interest is the leading consumer advocacy organization giving the straight talk about the food industry in America. CSPI is one of the few sources for hard-to-find information—like what exactly goes into that appetizer at your favorite chain restaurant.

Glycemic Index
www.glycemicindex.com
The glycemic index is a ranking of foods according to the rate at which they become converted to glucose in your blood. Visit this site for a directory of glycemic index values in common foods, compiled by the Australian researcher who first developed the scale.

The Okinawa Diet Program
P.O. Box 52287
311 16 Ave NE
Calgary, AB T2E 8K9
Canada
www.okinawa-diet.com
The Okinawa Diet is a low-calorie diet advocating whole foods high in water and fiber. The plan offered at this subscription site may or may not be for everyone, but there are few who will

argue with the wisdom of eating foods less dense in calories, a subject the authors have investigated and categorized thoroughly.

Tufts University Health & Nutrition Letter
Subscription Department
P.O. Box 420235
Palm Coast, FL 32142-0235
(800) 274-7581
www.healthletter.tufts.edu
This site is home to the Tufts University Health and Nutrition Letter, a leading sounding board for research and information on food ingredients, nutritional arguments, food trends, and other news of interest in the world of nutrition.

STRESS, MENTAL HEALTH, SPORTS PSYCHOLOGY, MENTAL PERFORMANCE

Albert Ellis Institute
45 E. 65th Street
New York, NY 10021
(800) 323-4738
www.rebt.org
Albert Ellis is the psychologist most credited with having developed cognitive behavioral therapy, a logic-based approach to mood management that has its roots in Greek philosophy, and one of the few methods in all of mental health to have ample empirically based research demonstrating its effectiveness.

Association for the Advancement of Behavior Therapy
305 7th Avenue, 16th Floor
New York, NY 10001-6008
(212) 647-1890
www.aabt.org
The AABT is the organizing body for

cognitive behavioral therapists nation-wide, and a great starting point to locate one in your area.

Institute of HeartMath
14700 West Park Avenue
Boulder Creek, CA 95006
(831) 338-8500
www.heartmath.org.
HeartMath is a stress management organization researching the interaction between stress and mental functioning and performance. It counsels corporate and individual clients in a self-directed method of controlling stress in the moment by modulating heart rate variability, or the rate of change in the distance between heartbeats.

LGE Performance Systems, Inc.
9757 Lake Nona Road
Orlando, FL 32827
(407) 438-9911
www.corporateathlete.com
LGE Performance Systems is home to the sports psychology and performance improvement company led by Jim Loehr, a psychologist, author of the Power of Full Engagement, and innovator in observing the habits utilized by high-achieving athletes to stay alert and perform at their very best.

Reflective Happiness
www.reflectivehappiness.com
This website is run by Martin Seligman, a pioneering researcher in psychology and founder of the school of research into human effectiveness known as positive psychology. It's a great starting point for locating books and materials on the ways of effective, happy, and fulfilled people.

ADVENTURE TRAVEL

Away.com
www.away.com
Away.com is home to Outside Online and is a great site for exotic travel advice, connections, information, and opinions.

Backroads
801 Cedar Street
Berkeley, CA 94710-1800
(800) 462-2848
www.backroads.com
Backroads adventure travel company is an active touring organization offering fully prepared luxury biking and walking trips in scenic destinations around the world.

Mountain Travel Sobek
1266 66th Street
Emeryville, CA 94608
(888) 687-6235
www.mtsobek.com
Specializing in small group travel ranging from rafting to camel trips to safaris, Mountain Travel Sobek adventure travel company arranges active vacations in all corners of the globe.

TRAINING ARTICLES AND RESEARCH

Human Kinetics
P.O. Box 5076
Champaign, IL 61825-5076
(800) 747-4457
www.humankinetics.com
Human Kinetics press is a specialized publisher of fitness books on every subject, for every athlete.

Peak Performance

67-71 Goswell Road
London EC1V 7EP
United Kingdom
www.pponline.co.uk
Peak Performance online is a UK-based subscription newsletter that offers a litany of well-researched articles on training and a highly informed online support community for athletes.

GYMS

Airport Gyms

www.airportgyms.com
This is a great free locator of gyms either in or near airports, for those stuck on layovers.

TRAIL FINDERS

All American Trail Running Association

P.O. Box 9454
Colorado Springs, CO 80932
(719) 573-4133
www.trailrunner.com
The All American Trail Running Association provides written guides to running trails across the U.S.

Trails.com, Inc.

1501 Western Avenue, Suite 304
Seattle, WA 98101
(206) 286-0888
www.trails.com
Trails.com is a subscription service online guide to trail maps and information.

RACES

The Active Network, Inc.

10182 Telesis Court, Suite 300
San Diego, CA 92121
(888) 543-7223
www.active.com
Visit this site for online registrations for marathons and bike races around the country.

American Cross Country Skiers

P.O. Box 604
Bend, OR 97709
www.xcskiworld.com
Hosted by American Cross Country Skiers, this site is home to the American Ski Marathon Series and loads of valuable information on cross-country ski training and gear.

United States Adventure Racing Association

12403 Bluestone Circle
Austin, TX 78758
(512) 873-1205
www.usara.com
This site provides a guide to adventure races in the United States.

Urban Adventure Racing, LLC

(312) 464-3300
www.urbanadventureracing.com
This site is home to the Wild Onion and Wild Scallion urban adventure race series.

SELECTED BIBLIOGRAPHY

American College of Sports Medicine's *ACSM Fitness Book*. 3rd ed. Champaign, IL: Human Kinetics, 2003.

Baechle, Thomas, R. and Roger Earle, ed. *Essentials of Strength Training and Conditioning*. 2nd ed. Champaign, IL: Human Kinetics, 2000.

Benardot, Dan. *Nutrition for Serious Athletes*. Champaign, IL: Human Kinetics, 2000.

Birch, Beryl Bender. *Power Yoga*. New York: Fireside, 1995.

Blahnik, Jay. *Full-Body Flexibility*. Champaign, IL: Human Kinetics, 2004.

Bompa, Tudor O. *Periodization*. 4th ed. Champaign, IL: Human Kinetics, 1999.

Bompa, Tudor O. *Periodization Training for Sports*. Champaign, IL: Human Kinetics, 1999.

Brown, Lee E. and Vance A. Ferrigno and Juan Carlos Santana ed. *Training for Speed Agility, and Quickness*. Champaign, IL: Human Kinetics, 2000.

Burke, Edmund R. ed. *Precision Heart Rate Training* Champaign, IL: Human Kinetics, 1998.

Campos, Paul. *The Obesity Myth*. New York, NY: Gotham Books, 2004.

Carmichael, Chris with Jim Rutberg and Kathy Zawadzki. *Chris Carmichael's Food For Fitness*. New York: G.P. Putnam's Sons, 2004.

Chek, Paul. *Movement that Matters*. Encinitas, CA: The C.H.E.K Institute, 2000.

Clark, Michael A. and Rodney J. Corn. *Optimum Performance Training for the Fitness Professional*. Calabasas, CA: National Academy of Sports Medicine, 2001.

Fleck, Steven J. and William J. Kraemer. *Designing Resistance Training Programs*. 3rd ed. Champaign, IL: Human Kinetics, 2004.

Foran, Bill, ed. *High Performance Sports Conditioning*. Champaign, IL: Human Kinetics, 2001.

Gambetta, Vern and Gary Winckler. *Sport Specific Speed*. Sarasota, FL: Gambetta Sports Training Systems, 2001.

Harr, Eric. *The Portable Personal Trainer*. New York: Broadway Books, 2001.

Hsaiao, Hongwei and Petre Simeonov. "Preventing Falls from Roofs: A Critical Review." *Ergonomics*. April 15, 2001.

Loehr, Jim and Tony Schwartz. *The Power of Full Engagement*. New York: Free Press, 2003.

Laskowski, Edward R. "Snow Skiing." *Physical Medicine and Rehabilitation Clinics of North America*, Volume 10, No. 1 (1999).

Laskowski, Edward R., and Karen Newcomer-Aney and Jay Smith. "Proprioception." *Physical Medicine and Rehabilitation Clinics of North America*, Volume 11, No. 2 (2000).

Marieb, Elaine N. *Human Anatomy and Physiology*. 3rd ed. Redwood City, CA: The Benjamin/Cummings Publishing Company, Inc. 1995.

Musnick, David and Mark Pierce. *Conditioning for Outdoor Fitness*. Seattle, WA: The Mountaineers, 1999.

Pollock, Michael L. et. al. "The Recommended Quantity and Quality for Developing and Maintaining Cardiorespiratory and Muscular Fitness, and Flexibility in Healthy Adults." *Medicine & Science in Sports & Exercise*. Volume 20. No. 6 (1998).

Radcliffe, James C. and Robert C. Farentinos. *High Powered Plyometrics*. Champaign, IL: Human Kinetics, 1999.

Rolls Barbara and Robert A. Barnett. *The Volumetrics Weight Control Plan*. New York: HarperCollins 2000.

Sleamaker, Rob and Ray Browning. *Serious Training for Endurance Athletes*. Champaign, IL: Human Kinetics, 1996.

Van Raalte, Judy L. and Britton W. Brewer ed. *Exploring Sport and Exercise Psychology*. 2nd ed. Washington: The American Psychological Association, 2003.

Willcox, Bradley J. and D. Craig Willcox and Makoto Suzuki. *The Okinawa Diet Plan*. New York: Clarkson Potter, 2004.

INDEX